Chemo: Secrets to Thriving

From someone who's been there

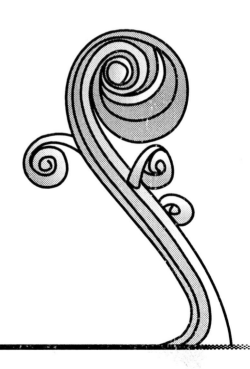

Written by Roxanne Brown
in collaboration with Barbara Mastej
and John S. Link, M.D.

Designed & Illustrated by Barbara Mastej

NorLightsPress.com
762 State Road 458
Bedford IN 47421

Printed in the United States of America

ISBN: 978-1-935254-53-9

Cover and book design by Barbara Mastej, Odd Man Out, LLC
www.oddmanout.biz

First printing, 2011

Dedicated to

the entire village it took to create this book,

including Dr. Link,

his new patient coordinator Stefany Montalbano,

and the Breastlink Medical Group;

Dr. Steiner and his assistant Susie Marble

at Saul & Joyce Brandman Breast Center, Cedars-Sinai;

my amazing psychotherapist Bunny Olds;

the Cancer Support Community; Healing Odyssey;

my fellow chemo travelers; Steve Brown,

and everyone else who

cheered us on during our quest to get this book

printed and on the shelves

for those who need it.

Table of Contents

iii • Dedication

vii • Forward

ix • Preface

x • Regarding our medical advice

xi • Introduction

2 • Pause, take a breath, and prepare for your journey

4 • Meet your new companions—they're here to help you

6 • Plan ahead and get organized

8 • Reach out selectively and ask for help

10 • Chemo and your kids

12 • Chemo, your job, and your rights

14 • Chemo and financial help

16 • Most people's number one concern—hair

18 • Don't flip your wig—get one FREE!

20 • How will I look after I get chemo?

22 • Chemo basics to handle BEFORE you begin chemo

24 • Have your calendar and notebook or journal ready

26 • A final checklist for the day before chemo

28 • Day of chemo treatment: first and subsequent infusions

30 • The day after your chemo infusion: preventing bone pain

32 • Right right right

34 • The days between chemo treatments

36 • Preventing infection and bleeding

38 • Steroid side effects: mood swings and weight gain

40 • Will I feel nauseous and vomit?

42 • Mouth and throat sores—how to prevent, alleviate, and stop them

44 • The hole truth and nothing but the truth about your orifices

46 • Now, here's the bottom line

48 • It's harvest time —

50 • Skin and nails —

52 • Regulating the toxic waste that comes out of you

54 • Flu-like symptoms: fatigue and anemia

56 • Rev up your energy!

58 • I just forgot what I wanted to tell you—all about Chemo Brain

60 • Feeling DEPRESSED

62 • Make a list of what helps you rise out of a downer day and then do those things

64 • Remember to be your own best friend and lighten your load

66 • Can you pass the forgiveness final exam?

68 • Post chemo highs and lows

70 • Rebirth and renewal

72 • About Dr. Link

73 • About the authors

74 • Acknowledgements

76 • Roxanne's favorite resources

79 • Roxanne's favorite supplements

80 • Roxanne's favorite books and publications

82 • References

85 • Tear-outs: shopping list, notes, and advice from your doc

*Chemotherapy for cancer is perhaps the most
feared treatment in all of medicine. Much of the fear is
based on older methods and preparations.
The good news is: major advances have been made
in both therapies and supportive care to minimize side effects.
One's life should not be on hold during chemotherapy.
On the contrary, it is possible to thrive during treatment.
This little book contains some wonderful advice on
how to achieve a better experience. Live well.*

—John S. Link, M.D.,
Breast Medical Oncologist
Oncology Medical Co-Director
Breastlink Medical Group

Preface

Not everyone with cancer is prescribed chemotherapy. This book is written for those who will take that journey. The unknown is often scary, even terrifying. I compiled this information from my own experience and the experience of many others, to educate and prepare you for chemo's potential side effects. Knowledge is power. After reading this book you won't be a victim of your treatment; you'll be proactive.

We're all different. Although some of the most common side effects are outlined in this book, please note **this does NOT mean you will necessarily get all, or any of them**. However, this guide prepares you with tips to prevent, alleviate, or stop many discomforts. ***The goal is to help you thrive—continue to enjoy life—throughout the chemo process.***

I was diagnosed with breast cancer just before my birthday. Nice present! During my illness I spent hours consulting oncologists, breast cancer survivors, books, magazines, support groups, newsletters, the Internet, and more. I was often frustrated by having to wade through long texts and multiple sources to find information. What I needed to know was scattered over this multitude of sources, plus even more fliers, handouts, and Xeroxed sheets from my nurses. I felt overwhelmed and disorganized.

After my treatment ended, I decided to create a simple guide from everything I learned (much of it from my collaborator Dr. Link), boiled down and in one place. This is the book I wanted to have—a book to help people manage side effects—a book to help people manage life as they go through chemotherapy. Barbara Mastej edited, designed, and illustrated the book to ensure it is user-friendly, with one spread per subject, easy to find topics, and illustrations to make you smile.

Although my personal experience is breast cancer, I believe anyone, male or female, who needs chemotherapy will benefit from this information. However, while I'm your friend and guide on this journey, I'm not a doctor. ***Always talk to your medical team. They know your particular type of cancer and your chemo prescription, medical history, and medical needs.***

Synchronicity and the koru

Our intention in creating this book is to share the many things I learned that may help you throughout the chemo process — physically, mentally and spiritually. When Barbara, who loves to garden, created the image of an unfurling fern frond for the cover design of this book, she envisioned it as a symbol of a fresh start.

The first time my oncologist Dr. Link saw the fern, he called it a *koru* and remarked it was perfect for this book. Barbara and I looked at each other and wondered aloud, "What's a koru?" Dr. Link's family happens to be from New Zealand. It turns out *koru* is a Maori word for the iconic spiral shape representing new life and new beginnings: growth, renewal, strength, peace, harmony, support, and loving protection. Perhaps Barbara's design was simple coincidence. I prefer to think it was something more.

***We wish you everything the koru symbolizes
as you take this step-by-step
journey through chemo.***

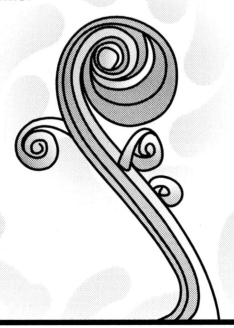

Chemo: Secrets to Thriving

From someone who's been there

Pause, take a breath, and prepare for

You probably picked up this book because you've been told you need chemotherapy. And you may feel stunned. I certainly did when it happened to me. I felt I had to rush. I told myself, "I've got to start this as soon as possible. I want to get this over."

In my case, my oncologist Dr. Link told me I didn't need to rush: I could pause, get other opinions—I got three total—look at options, and think about what I wanted to do with this news. He gave me good advice.

You may feel frightened. I did. I was especially fearful of nausea and vomiting. When I mentioned my worries to Dr. Link, he said, "We don't expect that to happen to you." Now, I was even more stunned. He said, "Lots of things can help you, like anti-nausea meds that go right in the chemo drip." Throughout chemo I didn't vomit and was able to nip nausea in the bud when it rarely and barely appeared.

Most chemo horror stories are based on things that happened 15 to 20 years ago when oncologists were using very few, very toxic drugs. Today many options and drugs are available, including supportive and complementary medicines as well as alternative therapies. Some are mentioned in this book.

your journey

You will find lots of help along this journey. You're not alone. Many people, places, and things can help make your chemo experience much, much easier.

Before you turn the page and begin meeting some of these people, places, and things, take a look at how far chemo has come by reading about Carol.

Carol's Exceptional Chemo Experience:
Carol and I shared the same chemo room. She is a parole officer and had 20 years on the job when she was diagnosed. She took six months off. Throughout chemo, Carol went to the gym every day and traveled extensively between her treatments—to London, Paris, Michigan and more. Her friends and family said they had never seen her so relaxed and happy—and she agreed!

Most of us land somewhere between a difficult time and Carol's experience. Once I learned the secrets in this book, I was able to enjoy my life while going through chemo. No, I did not go to the gym daily or travel abroad. I did take daily walks and enjoyed travelling locally.

By the way, do check with your oncologist if you are thinking of traveling.
Your oncologist will most likely want to prepare you for travel with special precautions and prescriptions.

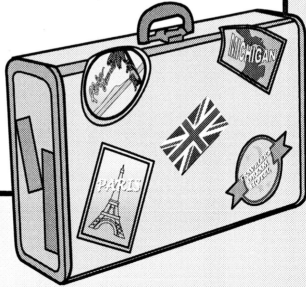

Meet your new companions—they're

YOU'RE PROBABLY FEELING A BIT OVERWHELMED RIGHT NOW. Although this is perfectly natural, a few things can help you overcome this feeling. *And they're available free if you can't afford to pay for them.* I highly recommend the following three resources (I affectionately refer to them as *companions*). These companions will help you take charge of your illness and regain a feeling of control. They create calm in what can feel like chaos.

WWW.CANCER101.ORG
1-646-638-2202
GET ORGANIZED!

www.Cancer101.org (1-646-638-2202) sends you an expandable file folder with dividers for pathology/test results, research, insurance, and more. You also receive a three-ring binder notebook (like a planner) with tabs for one-year calendar planner, medical history, appointment tracker, and more. All this costs only $18, but once again, it's free to anyone who can't afford to pay.

www.cancerandcareers.org sends the Living and Working with Cancer Workbook. This site offers several helpful booklets available to you. You can order the booklets or download them. Yes, they are free. The contents include legal rights, taking time off, returning to work, medical history, a health insurance claim payment log, and more.

WWW.CANCERANDCAREERS.ORG
KNOW YOUR RIGHTS!

here to help you

**WWW.FAMILYPATIENT.COM
EASY WAY TO COMMUNICATE!**

www.familypatient.com is a website that teaches you to build a FREE blog on their site. This is the easiest and most fun (yes, fun) way to communicate with concerned friends and family. Through your personalized site, friends and family can check on you by viewing the blog whenever they want. You can update when you feel like it, and you won't need to repeat the same news over and over. SEE IT TO BELIEVE IT. Go to familypatient.com. Click on Demo Patient—it's underlined in the body of text. Then click on SUBMIT under VISITOR LOGIN. Now click on Patient Update Reports at the top of demo page in a black box to see a sample blog. See how great it is! And, trust me, IT'S EASY and FREE.

CAREGIVERS

Many caregivers for older and younger patients may do the organizing, keep records, and track appointments, mood swings, and energy levels. They also communicate with employers, co-workers, friends, and family. These tools help you better plan the patient's life and your life while on this chemo journey.

WE HOPE YOU'LL THINK OF THIS BOOK AS YOUR FRIEND AND GUIDE. AND YOUR FRIEND AND GUIDE WANTS YOU TO PAUSE OFTEN ON THIS CHEMO JOURNEY. RESIST REACTING—PAUSE, TAKE A BREATH.

Think about it, sometimes you go so fast, you forget something important and you're required to stop for a "do over." Sometimes going fast actually takes longer.

Pause and take five minutes right now—I know you have five minutes—to call or log onto the Internet and get your companions on board for your chemo journey. This can be a long journey and you want them with you from the start.

I didn't know about these companions when I went through chemo. They would have made my journey much, much, easier.

Plan ahead and get organized

1.

Record and/or take notes with a friend when meeting with your medical people. Why? Because it's hard to remember what people say when you get the C diagnosis. Doing this prevents misunderstandings and phone calls back and forth. You may want a second and even a third opinion.

2.

Be discreet with whom you share the news. You may not want to be bombarded with phone calls, pitiful looks, and tales of who else had cancer and who survived and who died. If people start telling you this, you can say, "Stop, I don't want to hear it."

3.

Get a calendar Keep track of all your medical appointments or highlight them on your regular calendar. Why? Because when the insurance company and/or medical people ask when such and such procedure took place, you will know. Knowing what happened, and when, makes it easier to decipher medical bills.

4.

Don't panic, don't pay. Clarify your insurance coverage BEFORE getting procedures. Ask your insurance company to assign you a case manager, so you'll have one person to deal with on a regular basis. Don't panic when you get a medical bill, and do not pay immediately. Call the insurance company and wrangle with them about payment. Worst case—call your state insurance commissioner or contact your local media: newspaper/TV station.

VISIT WWW.CANCER101.ORG OR CALL 1-646-638-2202 FOR YOUR ORGANIZATIONAL TOOLS including notes, a file folder, a calendar and more. DO IT NOW!

5.

Go shopping
Get the supplements and supplies—such as your wigs, calendar, notebook—mentioned in here BEFORE your first chemo. Then you know you have them, which will help relieve anxiety.

6.

Keep a calendar, notebook, or journal
Keep a calendar, notebook, or journal. Record how you feel, both physically and emotionally once you start your first chemo cycle. This will most likely be your pattern throughout treatment. These notes will help you plan your life accordingly. For example, I was hyper and got a lot done the day before and after chemo, due to steroids. The day of chemo, I was out of it. Five days after chemo I needed two days of rest. In between, I needed a few naps during the day.

7.

Ask your oncologist about support groups
These exist one on one, in group settings, online, on the phone, and more. People who've gone through this experience can provide a wealth of information—like the suggestions I've included in this book.

8.

Create a laughter stash
made up of funny DVDs, books, CDs, and even a list of people who make you laugh. This is a great way to get away from it all and out of yourself. Laughter can be great medicine.

Reach out selectively and ask for help

You may be in shock when you get this diagnosis. My advice is to **pause and think before you announce to everyone you know that you have cancer**.

SHARE SELECTIVELY

This is what I chose to do so I didn't have to deal with sympathetic looks and endless questions from the entire neighborhood. You may resent people who say, "Everything will be okay." You may not want people to treat you as if you're fragile. By sharing selectively, I could be "normal"—not everyone was looking at me like I had the Big C. And the people I told were cool and supportive. If you want lots of calls, that's okay. I didn't want to keep repeating the same thing and telling the story over and over, so I used these ideas:

PREVENTING THE BARRAGE OF PHONE CALLS

- **Record an outgoing message** that thanks concerned parties for their call, and graciously lets them know you may not be calling back at this time, because you're a bit overwhelmed.

- You can **refer them to a website called www.familypatient.com**. You may log onto this site for free and post updates/news/photos/addresses to send cards to/when you want visitors/calls. Friends and relatives can check the website daily. You can make this personal and update when and as you wish. Recent studies show that blogging can help the healing process.

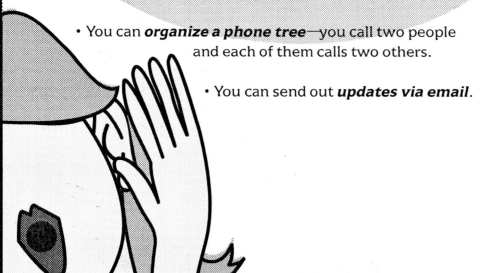

- You can **organize a phone tree**—you call two people and each of them calls two others.

- You can send out **updates via email**.

ASK FOR HELP—PEOPLE WANT TO HELP YOU
IT'S GRATIFYING FOR THEM

- *Ask as part of your update on www.familypatient.com.*
- *Set up a calendar* on *www.lotsahelpinghands.com* showing times you might need specific things, such as rides or help with tasks.
- *Be specific.* People do not know what you need, so be clear:
  - Can you give me a ride to chemo?
  - Can you send leftovers this way?
  - Can you prepare a meal for me/us?
  - Can you help me do light housekeeping, laundry?
  - Can you please pick this up at the grocery store, pharmacy, hardware store for me?

TELL YOUR FRIENDS AND RELATIVES THAT YOU'D STILL
LIKE TO BE INCLUDED IN REGULAR ACTIVITIES

If you're not up to it, you can always decline, but you'll have the option to participate. For me, continuing my regular activities in a modified version was therapeutic. I believe it contributed to my healing and a more positive outlook.

INSTITUTE THE HONESTY POLICY AND
KEEP IT FOR LIFE!

Be honest with people. Tell them "I may not return your phone calls. No, I don't want to go out. Please don't tell me about everyone you know who has had cancer. Let's just talk like we normally do. I want to go for a walk—do you? Can you help me with...?"

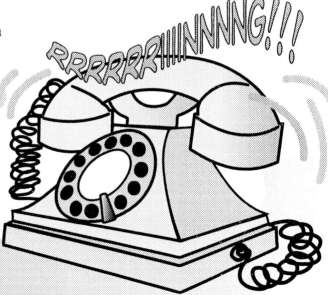

Chemo and your kids

They're watching you. So remember: how you respond to your diagnosis and treatment will affect how your kids react. No, this doesn't mean you must always be brave and stoic and never let on you're having a hard time. It's okay for kids to see you cry or be down and vulnerable. That's life, and this is how your kids learn about life. We aren't always happy. Things don't always go well. But despite that, we go forward, and usually a better, brighter day comes along.

Be truthful and at the same time KEEP IT SIMPLE and age appropriate with the information you give your kids. If you don't tell them what's going on they will make their own assumptions and conclusions, and that will truly be scary. You've heard how huge that monster under the bed can grow and what it can do. Clarify what's going on and what can be expected:

- Cancer is not contagious. ***Explain to them what it is and how it works.***
- Cancer is not anyone's fault—***definitely not their fault.***
- ***Do tell them what's going on.*** "My hair will fall out from the medicine. That's how strong the medicine is while it works to make me better. Later my hair will grow back, possibly better than ever—thick and curly."
- ***Do let them help you***—make art for you, tuck you in, bring you a glass of water.
- ***Do let them be involved in the process***—"Look what Mommy got as a gift from LOOK GOOD FEEL BETTER. We can play with this make-up." *LGFB* helps with and gives you free make-up.
- ***Do try to maintain a normal routine as much as possible***—pancakes on Saturday, a family movie at home on Sunday. If you can't go to a soccer game, maybe their favorite Uncle Fred can attend.

Spouses, caretakers, kids, and you, all need to be treated with loving kindness. It won't be perfect. And yes, you will still have fights and arguments. Duh, this is stressful. So I ask you to **PAUSE and THINK before you speak.** You probably won't always do this, so aim for progress, not perfection. Which reminds me, do **practice your spiel before you speak to kids** (and others, as a matter of fact, such as your boss, friends and co-workers).

Inform the other adults in your kids' lives about what you and your family are going through, so that they can be prepared to offer support.

Families and kids can get support at:
www.FamiliesCan.org
and www.KidsKonnected.org
or call
1-800-899-2866.

And remember, **you and your spouse—along with your kids—may all benefit from some professional help**.

NOW IS THE TIME FOR LOVE, LOVE, LOVE AND MORE LOVE, LOVE, LOVE...

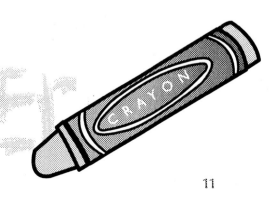

Chemo, your job, and your rights

Many people continue to work throughout chemotherapy. Others don't.
The folks I met in the hospital and in my support groups had varied approaches.

- One person I met said **she did not tell anyone at her job**.
  That's right—NO ONE.
- Another person had a wig made that matched her hair exactly.
  She told only her boss.
- Other people chose to **tell everyone** they knew.
- One woman said **her co-workers covered for her** when she needed time off
  and even **donated sick and vacation days** to her. She felt very blessed.
- My friend Laura told her co-workers and was then **asked to please take
  disability**, because she looked too "strange" (pale with no hair) to fit the
  firm's designer image. In the end, **she LOVED the time off**.
- A couple of people said that **they arranged for a flexible work schedule**.
- One woman **brought a couch into her office so she could take naps**.
  Another girl said she moved to an office closer to the bathroom.
- **Other people quit their jobs.** Some agreed to lay-offs and thereby collected
  severance and/or unemployment.

When it comes down to it, this is your call. Only you will know what's right for
you. ***www.cancerandcareers.org has lots of work-related information***,
including legal rights, taking time off, returning to work, medical history,
a health insurance claim payment
log, and more.

THE HEALTH INSURANCE PORTABILITY AND ACCOUNTABILITY ACT (HIPAA)

This act relates to **privacy rights**
regarding your cancer diagnosis and
treatment. It helps ensure health
insurance coverage and totability.

> **My story:** Since I was starting a new job, I initially told only my boss about my diagnosis and that I'd be going through chemo. After talking with other people and through experience, I learned to schedule my chemo on Tuesday, since I was good the rest of the week. Then I could sleep most of Saturday and Sunday. When I began to lose hair, I told my co-workers.

THE FAMILY AND MEDICAL LEAVE ACT (FMLA)

This act **protects employees' jobs at companies with 50 plus staff** for up to 12 weeks of unpaid leave with continuation of benefits and health insurance. **Caregivers are also covered under this act.** The law exists on both a state and federal level and differs accordingly. Here in California a neighbor of mine was able to take time off with pay to take care of her husband. Check with your employer to find out your rights. **If anyone (from the CEO on down) at your company has taken advantage of this law, they may have set a precedent—meaning you may be able to get the same benefit they did.**

THE AMERICANS WITH DISABILITIES ACT (ADA)

This act requires employers to make "reasonable accommodation" to allow employees to function properly in their job. It also protects employees from discrimination. If you find yourself experiencing discrimination during your chemotherapy, **talk to your supervisor, co-workers, human resources person, and medical team**. If you do need to pursue legal action, **KEEP RECORDS—tracking who, what, and whenever** something is said or done.

BE CREATIVE, RESOURCEFUL AND FLEXIBLE

It's helpful if you approach your employer, co-workers, and HR department with a clear notion of what is BEST FOR YOU. **Employers appreciate when you are flexible and solution-oriented** so you can get time off as needed, while they continue to have a cooperative and productive person on staff. **Try to make this a win-win situation.**

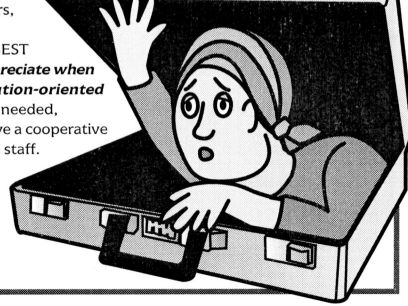

Chemo and financial help

You needn't panic over the financial aspect of chemotherapy. Help is readily available and it's just a matter of using the proper resources. Being pro-active is your key to success. ***Don't assume you make too much money to qualify for financial assistance.***

NATIONAL ORGANIZATIONS TO CONTACT:
- ***Cancer Care (www.cancercare.org—1-800-813-4673).*** Their website's ***Financial Help*** section provides comprehensive information and a fact sheet: Financial Help for People with Cancer. They also remind you to use your local elected officials if necessary. Talk to the people at Cancer Care. They care!
- ***The American Cancer Society (www.cancer.org—1-800-227-2345) and The National Cancer Institute (www.cancer.gov—1-800-422-6237).*** Apply to every program relevant to your needs.
- ***The National Cancer Coalition (www.nationalcancercoalition.org—1-919-821-2182)*** has a program that gives financial assistance to those in need.
- ***The Partnership For Prescription Assistance (www.pparx.org—1-888-477-2669)*** may get you help with the cost of medication.
- ***FamiliesCAN (www.familiescan.org)*** offers financial assistance for non-medical expenses.
- ***Contact charities*** affiliated with various religious groups.

LOCAL ORGANIZATIONS:
The Beckstrand Foundation—www.beckstrand.org, 1-949-955-0099 helps people in need who live in particular areas of Southern California. They paid two months of my friend Zita's family's health insurance premiums. On a national level they offer scholarships to people under the age of 25 who are going through cancer and want to attend college, or have already enrolled. Cool!

SOCIAL WORKERS
Talk to a social worker at each hospital where you receive testing or treatment. Ask all about financial assistance. Social workers are knowledgeable!

LIBRARIES
Ask your local reference librarian to help you find financial assistance resources. Librarians are trained to be amazing researchers.

EMPLOYERS

Please see section, ***Chemo, Your Job, and Your Rights*** on pages 12-13.

INSURANCE

Please see section ***Plan Ahead and Get Organized***, Point 4 on page 6.

BRAINSTORMING

Ask your friends for creative help. Start a registry so that people can gift you things you may need. Have a neighbor collect anonymous donations from other neighbors. Someone did this in our neighborhood and it worked. Your church, synagogue, or mosque can host a fundraiser. Your whole block might have a yard sale. Get your story in the newspaper. Now you're thinking!

VERY IMPORTANT

When you start to receive bills from your treatment facilities, call the billing department and business office. ***Ask them if a financial counselor or financial assistance is available. Apply promptly.***

Remember, you don't have to do all this research or fill out the forms yourself. Enlist friends and family to help.

Money is often a huge stressor. This list will help you begin finding relief. The resources section in the back has further options, and many more resources are available than we've listed. We hope this knowledge allows you to pause, breathe, and feel embraced by all the people and programs who want to assist with your healing journey.

Cancer Care sent Zita a check for transportation expenses to hospitals. Parking can add up. In her case, they also paid co-pays for chemo and many cancer-related drugs. This included many pills, such as anti-depressants and endocrine therapy. They also hooked her up with a professional therapist for weekly phone therapy sessions. **We love you Cancer Care!**

Most people's number one concern—hair

YES—FOR BREAST CANCER PATIENTS, HAIR USUALLY FALLS OUT FROM HEAD TO TOE.

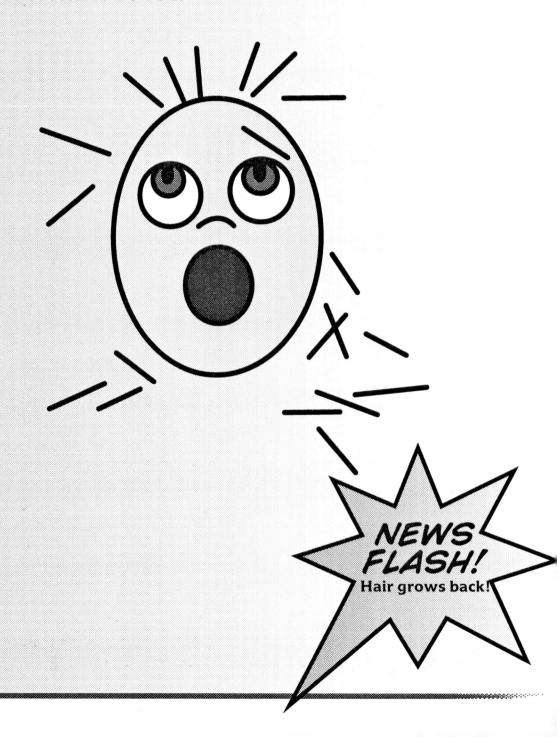

NEWS FLASH!
Hair grows back!

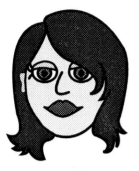

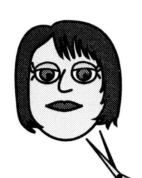

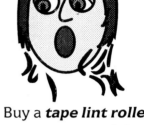

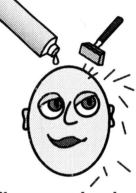

BE PREPARED.

1. Cut your hair short to chin length, so when it begins to fall out the event feels less traumatic.

2. Buy a **tape lint roller** or use tape to pick up the shedding hair.

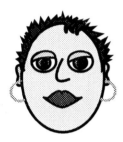

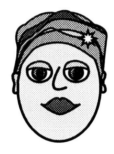

3. When it begins to fall out (for me this was 10 to 14 days after my first chemo) **cut it to one inch** and...

4. Go shopping for your wigs (scarves, hats, turbans, cotton nightcap) now!

5. Shave your head about a week after the one inch cut, or you may look like a forlorn kiwi.

6. After washing your bald head, spread **a dime size drop of conditioner** on it and leave it there. This prevents dry scalp.

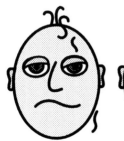

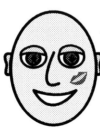

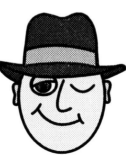

MEN JUST MIGHT LOVE THEIR NEW TRENDY LOOK.

Take a look around—**bald is hip!** Celebs like Kobe, Bruce, and tons of rock stars **shave their locks** to **enhance virile looks**.

17

Don't flip your wig—get one FREE!

Ask your oncologist to write a prescription for a hair or cranial prosthesis and you may be able to get a wig FREE. Various organizations often offer free wigs—talk to the American Cancer Society. If you buy your own, they cost from 99 cents on eBay to thousands for human hair (no need—for me, synthetic was better and cheaper). I spent from $20 to $60 and got lots of compliments on my "hair."

WIG WHEREABOUTS

Ask your medical people or the American Cancer Society. Check the Internet, catalogues, wig stores and others such as costume stores. Talk to people who do plays—and more. Talk to your oncologist. Do research.

WIG ADVENTURE

I got several wigs and enjoyed the different colors, styles, and personalities.

WIG INCOGNITO

If you prefer, you can get a wig that closely matches your own hair, or have one made.

WIG OUT

My adventurous friend Annie got Medusa wigs with snakes, Raggedy Ann wigs, and feather wigs. She had lots of fun.

THE LONG AND THE SHORT OF IT:

- Your wig will **keep your head cozy** in the winter—you won't need a hat.

- **Synthetic wigs are cheaper and easier to maintain** than real hair wigs

- Use **a metal hairbrush to comb a synthetic wig** to prevent static—about $1.

- **To store a wig, turn it inside out.** Shake it out before wearing.

- To curl or style your wig, **use styrofoam rollers**. Excess heat may melt it.

- It's okay for you or your stylist to **trim your wig**.

- **Wash your wig with regular or wig shampoo** when it needs cleaning—every 2 months. Wearing a paper towel under it keeps it cleaner.

- **Swish the wig around in the sink** with water and shampoo, then rinse and blot dry.

- Shape the wig by putting it on your head or a styrofoam head—about $5.

- **Don't comb the wig while it's wet**, the shape may go bye-bye.

COMMON SYNTHETIC WIG SENSE

WEAR A PAPER TOWEL UNDER YOUR WIG. THIS WORKS! You'll be comfortable & your head will stay cooler.

WHEN WILL MY HAIR COME BACK?

Approximately three months after my last chemo, my hair was about one inch long and was thick enough to style and color. At that time, you can Use a teeny **dab of hand lotion** to give this hair texture, volume, and shine. It works!

How will I look after I get chemo?

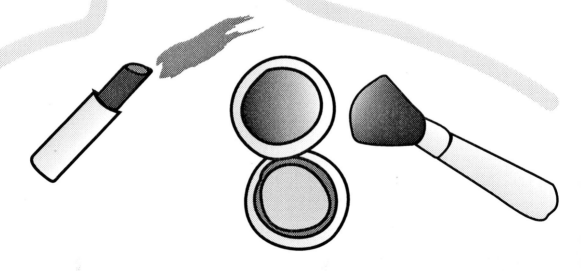

"LOOK GOOD FEEL BETTER"
is a FREE SERVICE that offers
instructions on using make-up,
wigs, scarves, and more during
this awkward time.
Contact them at:
www.LookGoodFeelBetter.org
or
1-800-395-LOOK.

They often give you great
makeup— free! Thank you LGFB!

IF THIS SERVICE IS NOT IN YOUR AREA:
- Ask a makeup artist at a makeup counter
  to help you.
- Ask a friend who loves makeup to help you.

EYEBROW LOSS:
- Pencil them in with short strokes.
- Use a medium or neutral color to look more natural.
- Wipe your mascara wand over that.
- And/or wear a wig with bangs.

EYELASH LOSS:
- Use eye shadow and liner.

WHEN CHEMO IS OVER
If you want to help those eyelashes grow in faster, thicker, and longer, use a stimulant containing a prostaglandin-like compound. I used RevitaLash®, although many similar products are on the market. I brushed this along my lash line and eyebrow line every night. It worked! This compound may have side effects, so be sure to read the warnings and get your doctor's approval. It can also be expensive, so ask your oncologist for a sample (as I did) or ask your friends to chip in as a "Goodbye Chemo" gift for you. Now my lashes and brows look better than ever.

LOOK MA—NO WRINKLES.
If you're taking steroids, they may give you a side effect called "moon face" meaning they will create a rounder, puffier face. This too shall pass once you stop chemo. Meanwhile, our wrinkles are puffed out—not necessarily a bad thing.

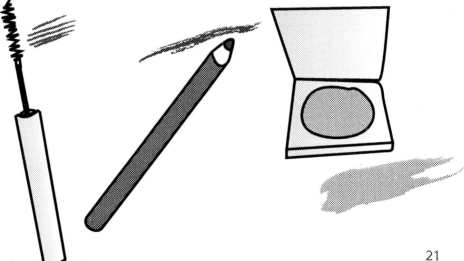

Chemo basics to take care of BEFORE

 TEND TO YOUR TEETH
Due to the possibility of infection, *you can't have dental work while undergoing chemo*. Get your teeth cleaned and dental work done before chemo.

 GET YOURSELF INTO THE STIRRUPS
Also *get a pap smear*.
(Now, how bad can chemo be?)

 HARVEST EMBRYOS, EGGS, AND SPERM IF YOU'RE CONSIDERING HAVING A FAMILY.
Discuss sex, fertility, and pregnancy with your oncologist. Discuss protecting the future fertility of children/adolescents getting chemo.

 NO ANTI-OXIDANT SUPPLEMENTS DURING CHEMO.
They may decrease chemo's effectiveness. Discuss with your medical team what you can and cannot take.

 PURCHASE MEDS, SUPPLEMENTS, AND OTHER THINGS YOU MIGHT NEED BEFORE CHEMO.
This lessens anxiety, because you'll be certain you have things to help you cope with side effects if they occur. First make sure your doctor has approved them.

 START YOUR MOUTH SORE REMEDY NOW!
See page 42. Mouth sores and sore throats are common. With the approval of your doctor you can find remedies to help prevent, alleviate, or stop them.

you begin chemo

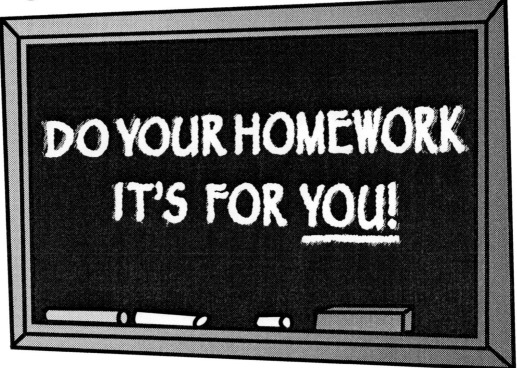

COMMUNICATE!

- *Discuss your fears and concerns with your medical team NOW.*
  I was worried about nausea. They put anti-nausea meds in my
  chemo mix and I used remedies in this book.
- *Tell staff about your sensitivities or allergies NOW* so they
  don't become an issue later.
- *Tell your doc and nurses what supplements and meds you
  are taking* as this can affect your chemo cocktail. They may not
  even want you to take aspirin—so check!
- *Ask for help if you feel anxious or aren't sleeping.*
  Your oncologist can prescribe anti-anxiety meds and prescription
  sleeping pills.
- *Inform staff which arm had lymph nodes taken out* and give
  that arm a break from blood work and IVs. Use the opposite arm.
- *Ask what will be in your chemo cocktail* (and write it down)
  to verify this at IV time.

Have your calendar and notebook or

FOR RIGHT NOW...
- *Get your chemo schedule.* Mine was Tuesday at 10 a.m. every three weeks.
- *Find out how long you will be in your first chemo.* The first one may be lengthy. Mine took six hours, because they put in the chemo slowly in case I had a reaction. That way, they could nip it in the bud. They were being cautious. HURRAH! My later chemo sessions were much shorter.

YOUR CALENDAR
Get a calendar to *record appointments and procedures so you'll have these dates for insurance billing and a general medical knowledge of what happened when*.

YOUR NOTEBOOK
or journal is for *recording your energy, moods, emotions, and the amount and type of pills you're taking*. This will help you work with the medical team to adjust your meds, if necessary. Recording your sleep and nap times and your energy levels will help you budget energy and plan your activities.

CONTACT CANCER 101 FOR AN ORGANIZATION SYSTEM
Visit www.cancer101.org or call 1-646-638-2202 to obtain items you'll need to keep track of your chemo schedule, insurance, and more.

PURCHASE A DAILY PILL BOX OR DOSETTE BOX
This will *help you remember to take pills*, because with chemo brain things can get fuzzy. For a particularly complicated pill routine, buy a dosette box that helps organize meds by time and day. It's extremely helpful.

VISIT THE CHEMO ROOM SO YOU KNOW WHAT TO EXPECT:
- *See what it looks like* and what food or water is provided. When you go for your infusions you may want to bring a plant, blanket, food, book, music, laptop computer, iPad, knitting, or games to make you more comfortable.
- *Observe a chemo IV going through a vein and a port.*

journal ready

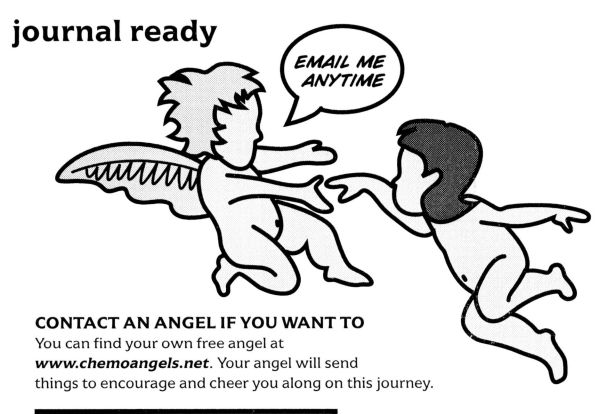

CONTACT AN ANGEL IF YOU WANT TO
You can find your own free angel at
www.chemoangels.net. Your angel will send
things to encourage and cheer you along on this journey.

NOTE: **Before your first chemo
you may want to attend a
support group or talk with
a person who's experienced
the same thing you're
about to go through.**
That's how I got my nausea remedy.
Anytime I felt the slightest nausea,
I took the remedy and was
instantly okay. This one helpful tip
made it worthwhile to meet Meryl,
my "bosom buddy." She had the
same type of cancer I had and was
seven years beyond the diagnosis.

**NOW YOU CAN GO TO
YOUR FIRST INFUSION—
PREPARED!**
Remember, preparation is more
than half the secret to thriving and
you are doing that by reading this
book. *I thought chemo would be
terrible. But guess what—it has
come far.* And once I learned the
secrets in this book I only encountered a few annoying side effects.
I was able to carry on with my life.
I wish the same for you!

A final checklist for the day before chemo

1. *Have you called 1-646-638-2202 or visited www.cancer101.org—*

for your organization kit?

2. *Have you taken whatever meds* you need to take?*

- Steroids
- Mouth sore prevention (See page 42)
- Always check with your doctor

3. *Do you have meds, remedies, and supplements your doctor approved—*

such as items for possible bone pain, nausea, or mouth sores?

(See pages 30, 40 and 42.)

4. Are you updating your calendar with the dates and times of procedures?

You will refer to this record often for insurance purposes and to answer questions from doctors, surgeons, radiologists, and others.

5. Do you have your journal

to record your energy, emotions, and moods during this journey?

6. Have you set up your FREE blog

at www.familypatient.com?

> * Some meds may be taken several days before chemo. Eventually my steroid regimen started three days before chemo. You may want to have things written down, taped on a mirror. I had the bone pain, steroid, and mouth sore remedies taped to the bathroom mirror. Plus I had my pill box. This helped me remember what I needed to take, and when.

Day of chemo treatment: first and subsequent infusions

Okay, you're going to report for your first infusion. Here you go—

- ***Dress in layers.*** The chemo room is often cold, so bring socks, a sweater, etc.
- ***Bring a hand-held fan*** if you are a hot flash lady.
- ***Bring anything that may brighten your space.***
- ***Bring your anti-nausea remedy and use it.*** Mine was salty pretzels and ginger ale. Alert staff the second you begin to feel nauseous, because it's easiest to remedy at this point. Always try to nip discomfort in the bud.
- ***Bring snacks, lunch, a computer, water, books, magazines, an iPad, knitting***—anything to help pass the time in what may be a long process. You might want to put together a special music mix for your chemo sessions.

COMMUNICATE WITH STAFF:
- Tell them about any allergies and sensitivities you have.
- Know which arm had lymph nodes removed—use the opposite arm for IV/blood work.
- Double check what chemo cocktail they're putting in your IV.
- Tell them how you are feeling. If the IV stings a bit, they can slow it down.
- Let them make you comfortable.
- Tell them if you feel any pain or nausea. Sometimes simply slowing down the chemo drip can lessen nausea.
- Find out what you should not be doing, eating, or taking.

- ***Network*** with people in the chemo room. Ask about remedies, but ***always check with staff/oncologist/nurse to get their okay***. Who knows? You could find a job. Or a good place to buy wigs. You might even find a new friend.
- ***Monitor*** your blood levels. The nurses will take blood for a CBC (complete blood count). If your red blood cells or white blood cells are low, they will help you remedy that. You can also eat food that's high in iron to raise the red blood cell count and/or take a non-constipating iron supplement.

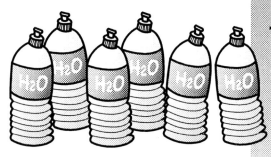

**TAKE IT EASY AFTERWARDS—
CHEMO DAY is NOT the day
to clean house, work, or
catch up on projects.
This is a day to take it easy,
rest, or watch TV.
DO REWARD YOURSELF
AFTER CHEMO.
Share a good lunch with
a friend or family member.
Do something that
brings you pleasure!**

- ***Drink water! Drink water!
  Drink water!*** You want to
  flush your system out and
  flush the chemo through.
  You don't want to dehydrate.
  Try to drink six 16 ounce
  bottles of water per day.
  These are the average size
  plastic water bottles you
  see all over the place.

- ***Pee, pee, pee!*** Yes,
  you can do this
  while getting
  your infusion
  in the chemo
  room. You want
  to wash all
  those nasty
  cancer cells
  away and out!

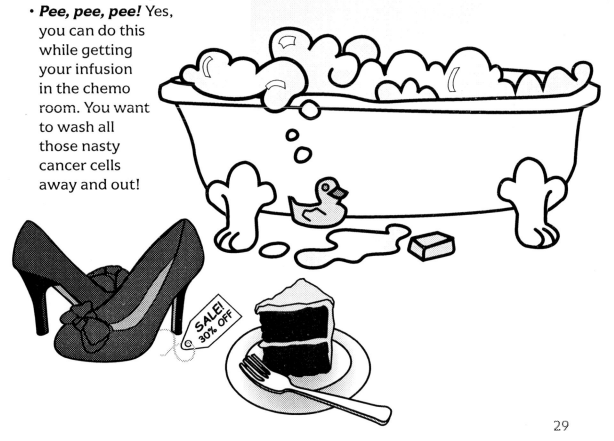

The day after your chemo, you may get a shot of pegfilgrastim (Neulasta®). The following remedy may help manage a common side effect—*bone pain*.

Talk to your doctor and try this remedy only with his approval. Pegfilgrastim is prescribed to increase your white blood cell count, which helps prevent infection. **Be sure the nurse warms the preparation in the palm of her hand before giving it to you.** Then it won't sting. My nurses didn't want to scare me by telling me I might experience bone pain from it later. I understand but disagree. I'm telling you up front.

30% of people who take pegfilgrastim get bone pain.

HALLELUJAH! AN UNEXPECTED (WELCOME) SIDE EFFECT FROM AN OTC DRUG HELPED ALLEVIATE AND STOP MY BONE PAIN. Patients at Breastlink found that when they took **Claritin-D® 12-hour** for their runny noses, their bone pain subsided. So **with Dr. Link's approval**, I took it every 12 hours (I had a runny nose from chemo anyway) the day of my shot and for two days after my shot. This worked for me. Maybe it's the placebo effect, but hey, it worked. **Again, get an okay from your doctor before trying this, since it may not be safe in your particular case. Some antihistimines can be dangerous for certain people, especially if you have high blood pressure.**

My doctor also told me he could prescribe a pain killer, such as a prescription dose of Advil® Ask your doc what you can do.

My advice is **discuss the possibility of this side effect with your doctor**. **DO NOT WAIT** until you're curled into a ball on the living room floor like Ms. Midwestern Grin and Bear It (me)! **There are ways to prevent, or at least alleviate, bone pain.**

If your doctor approves your use of Claritin-D® 12-hour, please purchase it before you get your pegfilgrastim (Neulasta®) shot. My friend Bobbi is no wimp. She's a longshoreman. When she began to experience bone pain she took a prescription pain killer, but it didn't help. Luckily, I sat next to her in the chemo room and told her about my experience with Claritin-D®. So she called her doctor, got the okay, and had her son run out to get it. She felt almost immediate relief. She is eternally grateful to me, her doctors, Breastlink, and Claritin-D®. Remember, not everyone can safely use this medication.

Another friend in my support group heard people talk about bone pain and decided not to take the shot. She got bronchitis. Chemo and bronchitis? No thanks!

NOTE: In my case, the bone pain was the worst side effect—mainly because I let it continue. It started slightly on Friday, grew worse on Saturday, and then became intolerable on Sunday. AGAIN, at the first hint of pain, talk to your doctor or nurse. The second worst side effect, for me, were the steroid mood swings I talk about later. Once these two issues were under control, it was all just an annoyance. Sure I was more tired than usual, needed some naps, and slept ten to twelve hours most days. But I continued to work, go out to plays, attend social events, and see friends and family. Yes, I had less energy and limited major events to one a day (shop, movie, dinner out, or work) but I felt good doing regular activities in moderation. Again, I believe participating in my normal life was immensely healing for me.

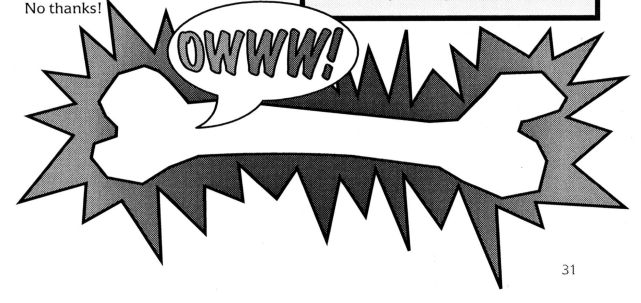

Right right right!

ASK THE RIGHT PERSON THE RIGHT QUESTION AT THE RIGHT TIME. THIS MAY BE THE MOST IMPORTANT SECTION IN THIS BOOK—READ IT!

When I began to feel stiff, I called my medical office and asked the receptionist, "Is this normal? I feel stiff and it doesn't feel good, but I suppose everyone feels that way." She answered, "A lot of people feel that way, but let me transfer you to the nurse practitioner." I said, "No, that's okay." When she insisted, I once again said, "No, I'm sure it's normal for chemo." Then I hung up. Am I a doctor? NO!

That evening I experienced severe pain; yet it was completely avoidable. I should have asked the right person—in my case the nurse practitioner.

I needed to ask the right person the right question. "This bone pain is increasing. What can I do?" The nurse had remedies for me, based on my particular medical history. Instead, I wound up in severe pain, calling my doctor in the middle of the night to get his advice for my particular case. Then, I got relief.

I needed to ask the right person the right question at the right time. In my instance, this should have occurred when I first began to feel weird. Relief was available. I didn't need to suffer.

We know when something is wrong. *Listen to your inner voice. Don't be shy. Don't think you're being a baby. Don't be afraid of imposing.* Don't take the WRONG PERSON's advice as I did in our Steroid Side Effects section. Your medical team's job is to help you. They want to help you. They are paid to help you. It is easier for them, for you, and for everyone if you nip things in the bud.

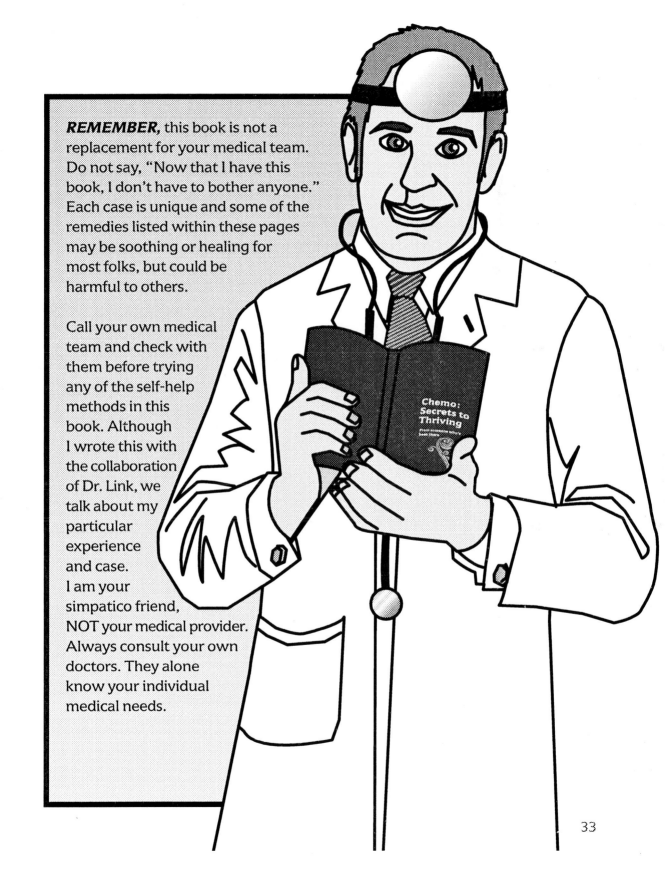

REMEMBER, this book is not a replacement for your medical team. Do not say, "Now that I have this book, I don't have to bother anyone." Each case is unique and some of the remedies listed within these pages may be soothing or healing for most folks, but could be harmful to others.

Call your own medical team and check with them before trying any of the self-help methods in this book. Although I wrote this with the collaboration of Dr. Link, we talk about my particular experience and case. I am your simpatico friend, NOT your medical provider. Always consult your own doctors. They alone know your individual medical needs.

The days between chemo treatments

- *Drink water, drink water, drink water*—at least four 16 ounce bottles a day.
- *If you don't like water, drink liquids.*
- *Avoid alcohol and caffeine*—they are dehydrating.
- *Pee, poop and sweat* to get toxins out.
- *Remember to take your meds and use the mouth sore and bone pain remedies* if needed.
- *Keep a journal* of how you feel, for yourself and your medical team.
- Discover and *record your pattern, then plan activities accordingly*.
- *Immediately notify your medical team if you experience pain* or any other side effect.
- *Monitor your temperature each day.* Call your doctor if it is at or above 100 degrees F (37.7 degrees Celsius) .
- *Eat more protein*—at least one more serving a day, such as an extra chicken breast or whey powder in your cereal. This boosts your energy, immune system, healing, and strength.
- *Eat five servings of fruit and veggies every day*—How much is a serving? A good rule of thumb is one fistful equals one serving.
- *Exercise moderately*—that might be a walk or stretching in your living room.

YOU WANT TO EAT MORE PROTEIN AND DO MODERATE EXERCISE BECAUSE CHEMO CAN WEAKEN YOUR MUSCLES. THESE TWO THINGS BUILD MUSCLES. SO DO THEM!

KEEPING YOUR LOG TO PREDICT YOUR FUTURE:
You want your log to reflect your energy/moods/emotions.
In addition to that, you can record:
- *your temperature*
- *blood counts from chemo visits*
- *your pills, how many, and when you're taking them* so they can be adjusted if needed.
- *the contents of your chemo cocktail* so you can double check and adjust if needed. My first chemo cocktail contained plenty of diphenhydramine (Benadryl®). I immediately fell into fits of laughter and then dropped off to sleep. Next time they halved the Benadryl. Darn!

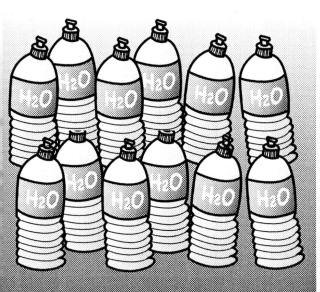

DRINK WATER!
DRINK WATER!
DRINK WATER!

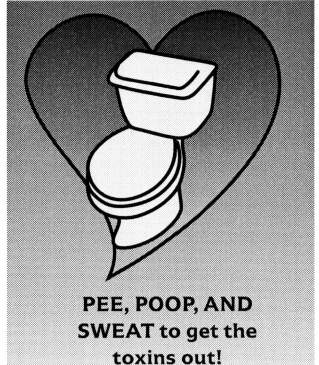

PEE, POOP, AND SWEAT to get the toxins out!

A SAMPLE LOG:
Day before chemo felt hyper and happy after taking steroids; took prescription sleeping pill at bedtime.

THE LOG CAN HELP YOU COMMUNICATE WITH YOUR MEDICAL TEAM AND HELP YOU KEEP TRACK OF THINGS. SO DO IT!

Preventing infection and bleeding

TAKE EXTRA PRECAUTIONS TO PROTECT AGAINST GERMS

Whether you are taking pegfilgrastim (Neulasta®) or not to boost immunity, you still need to do everything possible to prevent infection. Chemo destroys both good and bad cells and **may lower your white blood cell count, making you susceptible to infection**. Therefore:

- **Wash your hands often**—hands carry germs.
- **Do not put your hands to your face, mouth, or nose.**
- **Avoid sick people**, coughing people.
- **Avoid large crowds.**
- **Add more vigilance** when choosing activities and places. This isn't the time to bait hooks or play touch football.
- **Avoid dirt, cat litter, dog poo, and cleaning such things as fish tanks and bird cages.** I know someone who was hospitalized three days due to an infection after cleaning the cat litter. Don't do it.
- **If you cut your skin, wash with warm water and soap immediately.** Use a disinfectant.
- **Do not eat raw or undercooked fish (sushi), seafood, meat, chicken, or eggs** as these may contain bacteria that can cause infection.
- **If you have an infusion port, keep it clean and dry.**

PLATELETS HELP YOUR BLOOD CLOT

Before each chemotherapy infusion, your platelet count will be measured. If it falls below a certain level, your medical team will work with you. **If you notice bruising, nosebleeds, or headaches, notify your medical team.** You could be at risk for bleeding. Here's what to avoid:

- **Never take any medicine without first checking with your doctor or nurse.** This means aspirin, acetaminophen, ibuprofen, or anything else.
- **Avoid alcoholic beverages.**
- **Use a soft toothbrush to clean your teeth.**
- **Clean your nose by blowing gently into a soft tissue.**
- **Take care not to cut or nick yourself** when using scissors, needles, knives, or tools. Men, you may want to get an electric shaver.
- **Take care not to burn yourself** when ironing or cooking.
- **Wear padded gloves** when you reach into the oven or pick up something hot.
- **Avoid contact sports** and other activities that might result in injury.

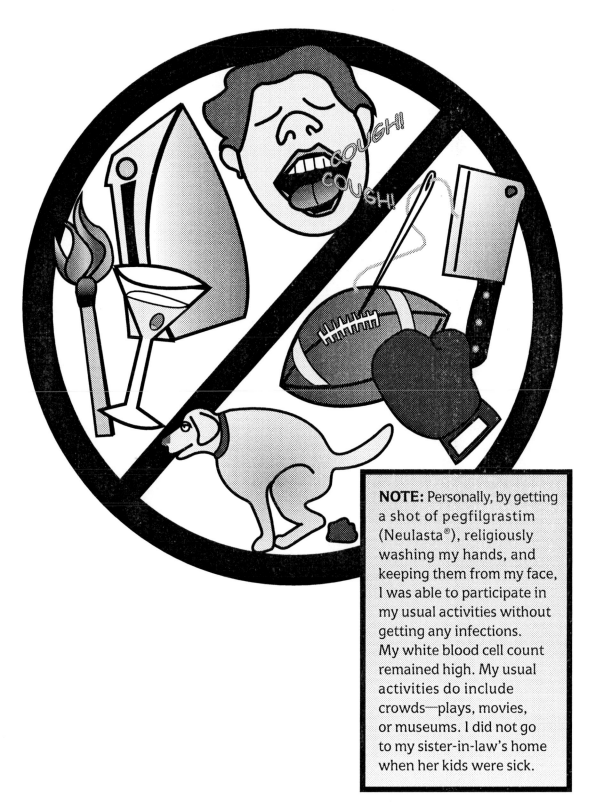

NOTE: Personally, by getting a shot of pegfilgrastim (Neulasta®), religiously washing my hands, and keeping them from my face, I was able to participate in my usual activities without getting any infections. My white blood cell count remained high. My usual activities do include crowds—plays, movies, or museums. I did not go to my sister-in-law's home when her kids were sick.

Steroid side effects: mood swings

Many people going through chemo receive steroids in their chemo cocktail and/or take steroids in pill form. I got both. No, you won't hit home runs, win the Tour de France, or be overcome with the desire to run a marathon. **Steroids may create intense mood swings.** At first I became maniacally happy and high, then experienced rage and anger, followed by deep depression and crying as I "came down" from them. **You don't have to go through this!**

WEAN YOURSELF ON AND OFF STEROIDS
WITH THE HELP OF YOUR DOC

My advice: Your doctor will start you on a regimen of steroids. The first dose is a starting place, and for me it was a big one. Steroids are prescribed to help prevent both nausea and fluid retention. Do discuss steroids with your doctor. If you are not experiencing much nausea or fluid retention, you may be able to take a lower dose of steroids. **This is where your journal will help you and your doctor create your own magic formula with the fewest possible side effects.**

OTHER STEROID-RELATED SIDE EFFECTS:
• They usually make people **a bit puffy**.
• Steroids sometimes **make your skin feel rubbery**.
• They **can make you ravenous**—I put on 20 pounds.*
• Steroids **may keep you awake all day and all night**.

A STEROID DO AND DON'T LIST:
• **Do create your own magic formula with your medical team.**
• **Do not diet.** Your body and brain need nutrition.
• **Do enjoy elastic waistbands**, pregnancy pants, and gym clothes.
• **Do eat more protein**—this builds muscle strength.
• **Do eat protein, veggies, and fruit** for energy and strength when you're ravenous.
• **Do not eat lots of junk food** like pizza and pie as I did when ravenous.
• **Do consider getting prescription sleeping pills from your doctor** such as Ambien® or Lunesta®.
• **Drink water! Drink water! Drink water**—flush the steroids through and out.

*Most people don't gain weight with chemo. My friends who ate more protein, veggies, and fruit did not put on weight. I could have avoided my 20 pound weight gain. At the same time, do not diet, because many people tend to lose weight with chemo. Your body needs nutrition at this time. Food is fuel for energy, immunity, and brain function—mind, body, spirit!

and weight gain

STEROIDS ARE ROBBERS, SO YOU MUST BECOME ROBIN HOOD

Steroids take calories from your energy stores and send them to fat cells. ***Don't eat too many sweets***, because sugar depletes energy as well. You get a sugar high, but then you crash. It's much better to ***eat protein, veggies, fruit, and complex carbohydrates***. These build strength, give you energy, and feed your body and brain. By the way, chemo reduces your metabolism. But take heart. ***I lost the 20 pounds once I was off chemo***, exercised, and stopped eating like a sumo wrestler.

My story:
In addition to the steroids in the chemo cocktail, I initially took several steroid pills the day before, the day of, and the day after chemo. I had the side effects noted above. So—dummy me—when I heard a woman in the chemo room say she only took one steroid pill, I decided to do the same—without checking with my doctor. I blew up like a pumpkin and began to choke on my tongue. I called the doc and, per his instructions, downed a bunch of steroids.
The lesson: Always work with your oncologist/medical team!

After I shrank back to my regular size, we experimented and tweaked my steroid regimen. The magic formula that worked for me was a gradual build up and decline of steroids over several days. This prevented me from taking that emotional roller coaster ride. I just rode the wave. This is my story, but we're all different. Do work with your medical team to find what's right for you.

Will I feel nauseous and vomit?

Some people experience a lot of nausea, while others have none. Many people are in between. I rarely had nausea. When I did, Meryl's Miracle (see below) worked for me. My oncologist also put anti-nausea meds in my chemo cocktail.

TO DO LIST:
- **Do talk to your medical team and voice your concerns regarding this topic.**
- **Do let them know the moment you begin to experience nausea**— because it's easiest to treat when it's just beginning.
- **Get prescription meds from your doc before your first chemo**—then you'll have them ready.
- **Have an anti-nausea stash** (I brought mine to chemo and kept it in my purse).

NAUSEA REMEDIES:
- **Meryl's Miracle**—salty pretzels and ginger ale
- **Ginger anything**—ginger tea or pickled ginger root (think Japanese)
- **Mint**—mint tea or fresh mint may help
- **Tea and saltine crackers**
- **Apple slices with tea**
- **Anti-nausea meds from your doctor**
- **Marijuana**—it works for some people when nothing else does. You can get a prescription from your doctor. It can be taken in pill form, eaten in baked food, or smoked in a cigarette, pipe, or water pipe. This may also help if you have a poor appetite.

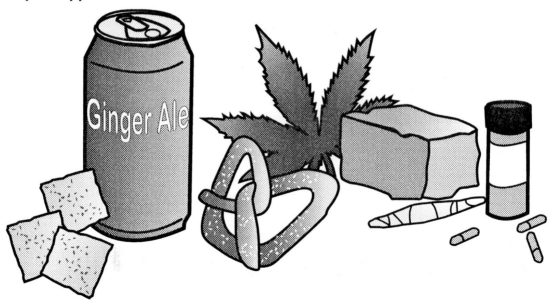

AVOIDING THE QUEASIES:
- *Eat and drink slowly.*
- *Avoid greasy, fatty, fried, and overly sweet foods.*
- *Drink liquids before or after a meal.*
- *If odors affect you*—microwave your meals, eat outside, eat foods that don't require heating, eat foods that have less odor, and stay away from strong scents like perfume and smoke.

RECENT STUDIES SHOW THAT ADDING GROUND GINGER OR GINGER ROOT TO FOOD DAYS BEFORE, DURING, AND AFTER CHEMO CAN REDUCE NAUSEA AND VOMITING.

IF YOU ARE VOMITING:
- *Let your doctor know* if you cannot keep food down.
- *If you're vomiting, carry sick bags with you* (like on an airplane). These are available online and at drug stores.

FOR LOSS OF APPETITE:
- *Try eating smaller amounts more frequently.*
- *Make food look attractive* with good china, cloth napkins and garnishes.
- *Make meal time a special and pleasant event* with nice music and china.
- *Experiment* with tastes, temperatures, and textures.
- *Cold or room temperature foods* may be more appetizing than hot food.
- *An alcoholic drink can stimulate the appetite* before a meal.
- *Drink supplements* like Ensure® and Boost®—with your doc's approval.

IF YOU HAVE A METALLIC TASTE IN YOUR MOUTH:
- Try using *plastic utensils or plastic/wooden chopsticks*.
- Follow the *mouth care guidelines* on page 42.
- *Chew sugar free gum* to mask the taste.
- *Drink plenty of water.*

Mouth and throat sores—how to

These painful sores are one of the main reasons I wrote this book. I found fellow patients at major, well-known hospitals/facilities did not know how to prevent mouth sores. Once their mouths began to swell with sores they tended to go into isolation and depression. Not good! Chemo affects the mucous membranes, thus creating this unsightly, painful side effect.

I STRONGLY URGE YOU to START the following remedy BEFORE CHEMO to PREVENT, AVOID, or ALLEVIATE MOUTH and THROAT SORES!

BREASTLINK'S MOUTH SORE REMEDY:
The first key to preventing and treating mouth sores is good oral hygiene.
- ***Brush your teeth with Arm & Hammer® Baking Soda and Peroxide toothpaste.***
- ***Use a soft toothbrush.***
- ***Floss regularly*** to prevent inflammation.
- ***Rinse mouth with baking soda, salt, and water or Biotene® mouthwash.***
- ***Drink at least four 16 oz. bottles of water daily***—a total of 64 oz. of water.
- ***Eat foods high in fiber.***

In addition to the above, with my doctor's okay, I started the following regimen one or two days before chemotherapy, continued it on chemo day, and kept going for three to five days after chemo:
- ***Glutamine Powder***—Add 10 grams once a day to 8 to 12 ounces of apple juice or Gatorade®. Swish and swallow for throat sores, or spit for mouth sores.
- ***Vitamin B6***—Take one 100mg tablet twice a day throughout chemotherapy to help the healing process of oral tissue.
- ***Lysine***—Take one 500 mg tablet twice a day for prevention of oral lesions.

This remedy worked for me. Always ask your doctor.
All things are not safe for all people.

prevent, alleviate and stop them

IF THIS DOESN'T WORK FOR YOU

If you've tried my remedy (with your doc's permission) and it doesn't work for you, talk to your doctor about the prescription drug Valtrex®. Or consider trying a couple of over the counter healing canker sore patches such as CankerMelts® and Canker Cover™.

When Susie from our focus group wasn't getting relief from any of these remedies, Dr. Link spoke with her dentist. They prescribed Valtrex® and an oral mouth rinse called, dexamethason. The combo cleared up Susie's problem. She says, "By taking Valtrex® and 1 tsp. of liquid dexamethasone, swishing, and spitting it out, my mouth sores were gone within 24 hours! Plus it tasted great!" You can see why it's important to consult your own doctor for a remedy designed especially for you.

My story:
I began using my remedy as soon as my mouth started feeling funny. This immediately relieved and eliminated the sores, and I continued using it throughout my chemo treatment. When chemo was over I went for a dental exam and got the best results ever—less plaque, no cavities, less deep pockets in gums! A great side effect!

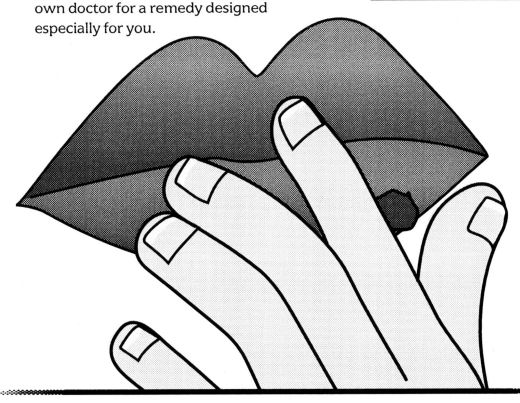

The hole truth and nothing but the

REGARDING YOUR MOUTH, NOSE, THROAT, EYES, VAGINA, PENIS—AND YES, YOUR RECTUM

MOUTH SORES—IF YOU DO GET THEM:
- *Skip the hot tea. Suck on a popsicle.*
- *Eat and drink foods at cold or room temperature.*
- *Avoid tobacco, alcohol, and mouthwash with alcohol.*
- *Use Carmex®* or something similar on the sores to soothe them.
- *If you feel a sore coming on, rub ice on that spot* and you may prevent it.
- *Rinse and gargle with 3% hydrogen peroxide.*

DRY MOUTH:
- *Use mouthwash and toothpaste specifically formulated to alleviate dry mouth*, such as Biotene®.
- *Sucking on a lemon or lemon drops may stimulate saliva*—only if you do NOT have mouth sores.

SORE THROAT:
- I had this side effect, but *the remedy on the previous page significantly lessened it*.
- *Drink hot tea with honey and lemon*—only if you do NOT have mouth sores. Very soothing!
- *Use throat lozenges.*

I generally experienced a combo of a runny nose and a dry nose.

RUNNY NOSE:
- *Antihistamines* such as Claritin-D®(but only with your doc's approval) will alleviate a runny nose.
- Keep small packets of soft tissues with you at all times.

truth about your orifices

DRY NOSE:
- *Use a moisturizer such as Vaseline,® Neosporin,® Aquaphor,® Vick's VapoRub® or Udderly Smooth® Udder Cream* to ease the dry tissue inside your nose.
- You may develop scabs inside your nose. Should you pick them and get a nosebleed that persists, *call your doctor or nurse and follow their instructions to stop the bleeding*. I had scabs and a little bit of blood, but did not get a nosebleed.

This double trouble may also manifest as a combo of runny eyes and dry eyes.

TEARY EYES:
- Keep those *small packets of soft tissues* handy at all times.
- *An antihistamine may lessen this.* Again, always read the packaging and check with your doc.

DRY EYES:
- *Talk to an opthomologist.*
- *Use natural eye drops.*

MORE SIDE EFFECTS INVOLVING YOUR EYES:
- *Your eyes may be extra sensitive to light. Be sure to wear a hat or visor and sunglasses with UV protection from the sun.*
- *Your eyesight may become temporarily blurry and/or deteriorate. If this occurs, let your doctor know.*
- *You may not want to change your eyeglass prescription until later*, because vision usually goes back to normal.
- *If your eyesight changes drastically, get a temporary prescription.* Don't put yourself at risk while driving or doing other daily and work activities. Invest in new lenses for the time being. Save your old lenses. They can be popped back into the frames when your eyes normalize.

Now, here's the bottom line

THE URETHRA, VAGINA, AND RECTUM:

More fun stuff. *Your urinary tract may become irritated and your vagina may feel dry, while your rectum gets moist.* Again, chemo affects mucous membranes and pH levels, therefore creating this combo effect.

Your urethra may grow thinner, causing your bladder to become inflamed. This creates an urgency to go to the bathroom (think yeast or bladder infection). Drinking cranberry juice daily helped alleviate this for me. And if that doesn't help, do talk to your doc; you may actually have a yeast and/or bladder infection.

Your vagina may become dry. You may want to use a water-based lubricant for sex such as K-Y® Brand Jelly or Astroglide®. Don't use oil-based creams or lotions as they can cause infection.

Your rectum may get moist and feel sore. Mine did. A few solutions:
• *Take a warm bath and thoroughly dry the affected area.* Some people recommended using a blow-dryer. Once it's dry, *put cornstarch or talcum powder on the area*.
• Another friend said her rectum felt dry and sore. She used *zinc and castor oil and Vitamin E to soothe it*.
• One friend's rectum bled. She called her doc. They gave her a suppository to stop the problem.

SEX LIFE...WHAT SEX LIFE?

What happens to a person's sex life during chemo? It depends on the individual. I have a friend who had a robust sex life throughout her chemo. I was not so interested. Men may find their penis at half mast (under the weather—at ease) during this time. Men, please talk to your doctor about your particular parts.

Breastlink's Dr. Link stresses **the importance of communicating your feelings to your partner and trying pleasurable touch without any demands**. He suggests asking for the physical contact you want, being specific, and tactfully setting boundaries if something does not feel comfortable at this time.

The good news is, you can still have a sex life, but if you aren't in the mood you don't have to use the old headache excuse. Once the long drought is over, sex may seem, well—sexier than ever. After chemo and radiation are completed you will likely have a renewed interest, as I did.

Dr. Link prescribed a vaginal suppository for me when I finished treatment. I used this three times a week. It moistened my vagina and my sex drive increased. Oh, and putting a bit of this same stuff on the outside of my urethra alleviated the urge to urinate. Other friends have used *Replens*®, *Gyne-Moistrin*® and *Lubrin*® for everyday vaginal dryness. These maintain vaginal moisture for one to three days, depending on the product. Always consult with your doctor.

Speaking of sex, let's move on to FERTILITY and MENOPAUSE.

It's harvest time—

**REGARDING FERTILITY FOR MEN AND WOMEN
WHO WANT BABIES:**

Chemo can put you into temporary or lasting menopause and/or sterility.* BEFORE chemo starts, discuss your fertility and options with your oncologist, others who have gone through this, and organizations that offer support:

- *www.myoncofertility.org is a wonderful site with resources, videos, animation, and more regarding cancer and fertility. Call 1-866-708-3378 for questions about fertility preservation options.*

- *Fertile Hope (now part of www.livestrong.org 1-866-673-7205) provides reproductive and fertility information and hope for people with cancer.*

- *Sharing Hope (part of Fertile Hope at www.livestrong.org) has a fertility preservation discount program.*

- *If you are pregnant at this time, you will find lots of information, support, and hope at www.pregnantwithcancer.org or 1-800-743-4471.*

Remember to **protect the future fertility of kids and adolescents** who are going through chemo!

**YOU MAY STILL NEED TO USE BIRTH CONTROL—
TALK TO YOUR DOCTOR**

For me, **menopause** meant hot flashes, mood swings, and a dry vagina that could be painful during sex. I got through it by:

- *Dressing in layers.*
- *Taking an anti-depressant/anti-anxiety drug.*
- *Talking to a psychotherapist.* Once you establish a rapport with the right therapist, you'll find yourself looking forward to these sessions about you.
- *Joining a support group.*
- Carrying a **hand-held fan** like the ones used by Spanish and Japanese ladies. This comes in handy for hot flashes or when you want to hide.
- Using **personal lubricants**—over the counter and/or prescription.

*Most women in their 30s do not lose reproductive capacity.

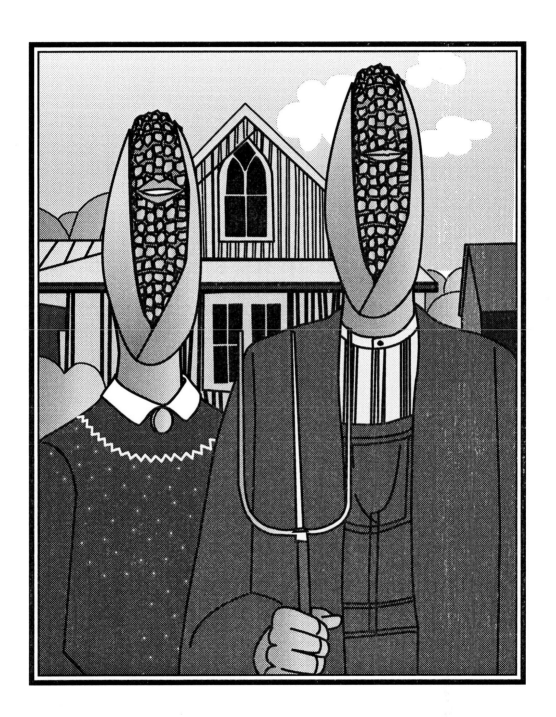

49

Skin and nails—

More than likely all of your hair will disappear. Yes, that too—no need for a bikini wax! You'll have hairless, smooth skin. However, you may also find yourself with dry, sensitive skin that feels kind of rubbery. Thank you, steroids.

DRY SKIN:
- *Baby your skin with gentle soaps* like Ivory®, Pears®, or Neutrogena®.
- I found *no need for underarm deodorant* once I had no hair there. If you want to use deodorant, try cornstarch, talcum powder,* or *Tom's® natural deodorant*. Think gentle.
- *Udderly Smooth® Udder Cream and Udderly Smooth® Extra Care Cream* are great for dry skin. The CHEMO PILL or infusion may cause redness, blistering, and peeling of hands and feet. These creams can prevent, alleviate, and restore skin health with your doc's Okay.
- Experiment. I would *shower, blot dry, and apply sesame or castor oil* on my skin.

DRY LIPS:
- Use *Carmex®, Vaseline®, ChapStick®* or other lip conditioners.

SUN SENSITIVITY AND DISCOLORATION:
Chemo and other meds may make your skin sensitive to the sun and cause darkening or discoloration. My arms became dark in some sections when not covered.

- *Cover up* when you go out in the sun.
- *Lavish sun block on every inch of your skin*—hands, ears, face—all of it.
- *Wear long sleeves and a hat*, wig, scarf, or other head covering.

*Remember NOT to use talcum powder on any part of your body during radiation. Also no deodorants containing aluminum.

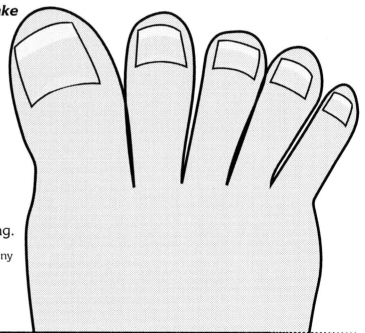

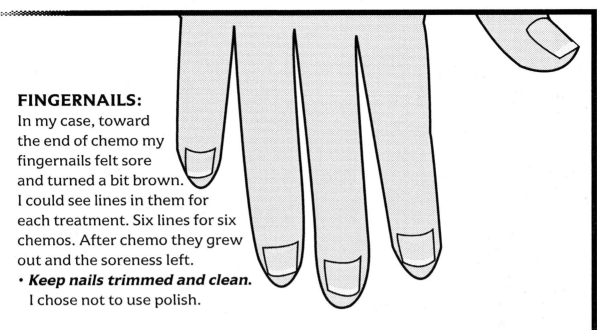

FINGERNAILS:

In my case, toward
the end of chemo my
fingernails felt sore
and turned a bit brown.
I could see lines in them for
each treatment. Six lines for six
chemos. After chemo they grew
out and the soreness left.

- **Keep nails trimmed and clean.**
  I chose not to use polish.

TOENAILS:

I had no problem with toenails, but my Bosom Buddy said hers fell out after
chemo was over. She wore shoes that covered them. And yes, they grew back.

- **Keep nails trimmed and clean.** Again, I used no polish, while others did.

MANICURES AND PEDICURES:

- **Pay attention to cleanliness and sterilization.** This is especially important
  if you go to a salon to have your nails done. Be picky about where you go.
- **Be careful not to cut your skin.** If you do, remember to immediately wash
  with warm water and soap and apply disinfectant.

TINGLES IN FINGERS AND TOES—NEUROPATHY:

Chemo can affect your nerve endings, causing **a feeling of numbness, pain,
or tingles in the tips of your toes and fingers. If you experience this tell
your doctor immediately**. Your oncologist may need to change your meds.
Additionally, here are tips that may quiet those "tips."

- **Vitamin B6 with calcium and magnesium** may help. My English friend was
  told to take 50 mg of water soluble B6, three times to four times a day. You
  pee it out. B vitamins are known to help your immune system and energy levels.
- **A footbath in warm water with hydrogen peroxide or oatmeal**
  can be soothing.
- **Acupuncture can be helpful as well.**

Regulating the toxic

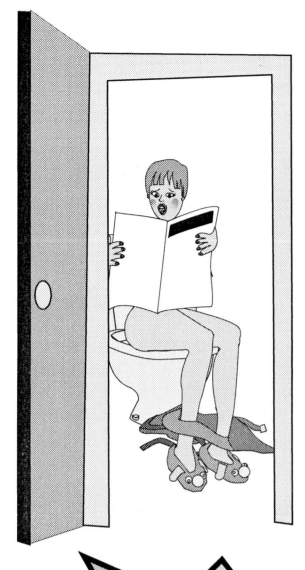

Yes, for the time being with all these chemicals running through you, **you are, in essence, your own toxic waste site**. My pee and poop DID smell like a toxic waste dump—no pun intended. I suspect even my sweat may have had a chemical odor. So be sure to:

- **Pee, poop, and sweat the toxins out.**
- **Drink at least four 16-oz. bottles of water a day.**
- **Do moderate exercise.**

CONSTIPATION:

- **Consult with your oncologist** on what you will use.
- **Do not take remedies/ meds/supplements** without first getting your doctor's approval.
- **Drink lots of water** and fluids.
- **Limit caffeine and alcohol**, which dehydrate you.
- **Eat high fiber foods** like oatmeal, prunes, and dried apricots.
- Try a few slices of **fresh ginger steeped in hot water** for 5 minutes, then add honey.

TIP:
I did use a natural laxative (with my doc's okay) that gave me a soft BM every day.

waste that comes out of you

DIARRHEA:
- *Avoid acidic and greasy foods.*
- *Don't drink with meals.*
- *Do drink lots of water between meals. Do avoid milk and milk products.*
- *Eat bland food like BRAT:* Bananas, Rice, Applesauce, and Toast.
- *Eat many small meals* throughout the day.
- *If severe, only drink clear, warm liquids and call your doctor ASAP.*

STOMACH CRAMPS:
- *Drink tonic water*—the quinine may help. Don't drink milk or milk products.
- *Massage* the area.
- *Move* around.
- *Swimming* may bring relief.

GAS AND FLATULENCE:
Yes, you may run on gas and putter around. I did this throughout my treatment. I told my pals about this "special" side effect and we all ignored it. They know your body is chemically active!
- *Try fresh mint tea or Colpermin® tablets* (with your doc's approval). Forget peppermint candy—too wimpy for this job.
- *Avoid gas producers: milk, beans, cabbage, etc., or ask your doc for anti-gas meds.*

HICCUPS:
- *Try breathing in and out with a paper bag* over your mouth and nose for 30 seconds.
- *Take a spoonful of sugar*, allow it to melt in your mouth, swallow.

BURPS:
- They happen. Let them come.

NOTE: I knew, and other people knew, I would fart, hiccup, and burp. We all accepted it. So what? That's the human body. On your walks you'll have a tail wind! At a crowded museum you can clear the room and have the exhibit to yourself.

Flu-like symptoms: fatigue and anemia

Low energy is normal during chemo, although I've known people who went to the gym every day throughout treatment. You may (and I did) experience flu-like symptoms. Your body is working overtime and will get tired.

STIFF AND ACHY LIMBS:
- *Stretch, walk, and do gentle yoga.* Exercise, movement, and stretching help relieve the stiffness.
- *If you have cramps in your legs, drink tonic water with quinine, massage them, and move around.*
- *Swimming may help.*
- If you feel dizzy, out of it, or off-balance, *be slow, conscious, and careful when walking*.

HEADACHES:
I often felt a slight headache when I was on chemo. An annoyance.
- Sometimes *just drinking two big glasses of water* will help
- *Only take something with your doc's approval.*
- My doc said NO ASPIRIN, but he allowed *Tylenol®, Advil®,* and *Aleve®.* So ask your doctor!

ANEMIA:
Although my white blood cells remained high throughout chemo and I didn't get any infections, toward the end of my treatment my red blood cell count did start going down.

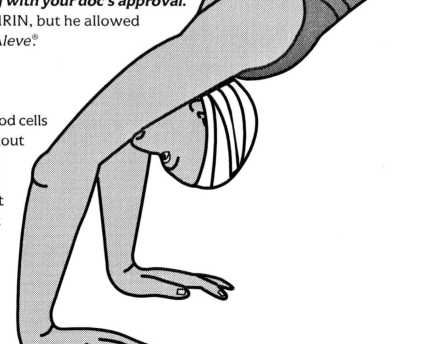

I already suspected this, as I had some of these **common symptoms of anemia:**
- **Shortness of breath**
- **Confusion/difficulty concentrating**
- **Dizziness/fainting**
- **Pale skin**
- **Rapid heartbeat**
- **Feeling cold**
- **Sadness and depression**
- **More fatigue and weakness**

THE ABCS OF YOUR CBC
- Red blood cells carry oxygen to tissues.
- White blood cells fight infection.
- Platelets assist in clotting blood and healing wounds.

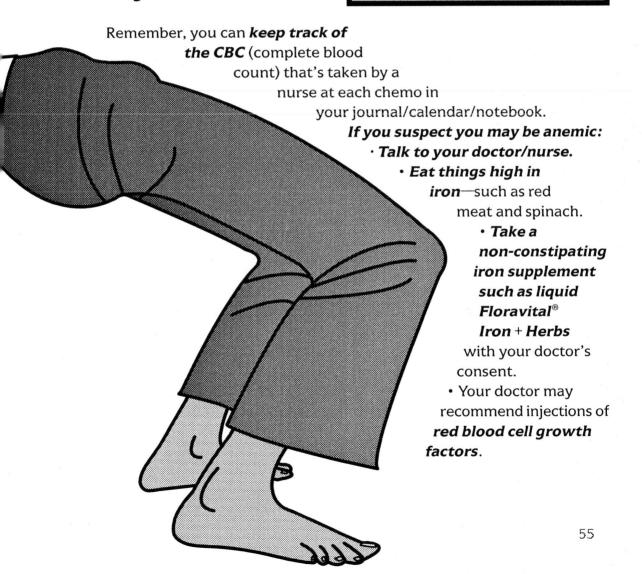

Remember, you can **keep track of the CBC** (complete blood count) that's taken by a nurse at each chemo in your journal/calendar/notebook.

If you suspect you may be anemic:
- **Talk to your doctor/nurse.**
- **Eat things high in iron**—such as red meat and spinach.
- **Take a non-constipating iron supplement such as liquid Floravital® Iron + Herbs** with your doctor's consent.
- Your doctor may recommend injections of **red blood cell growth factors**.

Rev up your energy!

EXERCISE GIVES YOU ENERGY:

This is a fact. Plus, you can **do this in your own home, or...**

- Ask your medical team, local Y, social service, or non-profit organizations about classes. **They're often free** to people going through chemo/cancer.
- If you've had lymph nodes removed/surgery, check with your surgeon/oncologist on how to exercise the arm/surgery area.
- Make any exercise/yoga/swim instructor aware of your surgeries, pain, injuries, and where lymph nodes were removed.
- **Get outside in the fresh air.** Get out of your house.
- **A simple walk can recharge you** both physically and mentally.
- **Put on some upbeat music. Do you love to dance?** Invite your kids or a friend and start moving. Make it fun and you'll forget you're exercising.

ACUPUNCTURE:

- **Your insurance** may cover this treatment.
- Training facilities often offer **lower charges**.
- **Teach yourself key acupressure points** from the Internet or library.

IRON:

- Be sure to watch these levels. When mine went down I felt tired and out of breath. Dr. Link recommended Florivital® Iron + Herbs, a **non-constipating supplement, plus foods high in iron**. Always check with your doctor to see if this is a safe option for you.

MORE WAYS TO HELP REBUILD YOUR BODY:

- **Fresh veggie and fruit juices** helped me. Some people stay away from these to avoid potential infection.
- **Eat plenty of protein** to help build muscle strength.
- **Take a Vitamin B complex** to help give you energy.
- **Drink water! Drink water! Drink water!**
- **LAUGH!** Laughing can increase circulation and exercise your skeletal muscles.

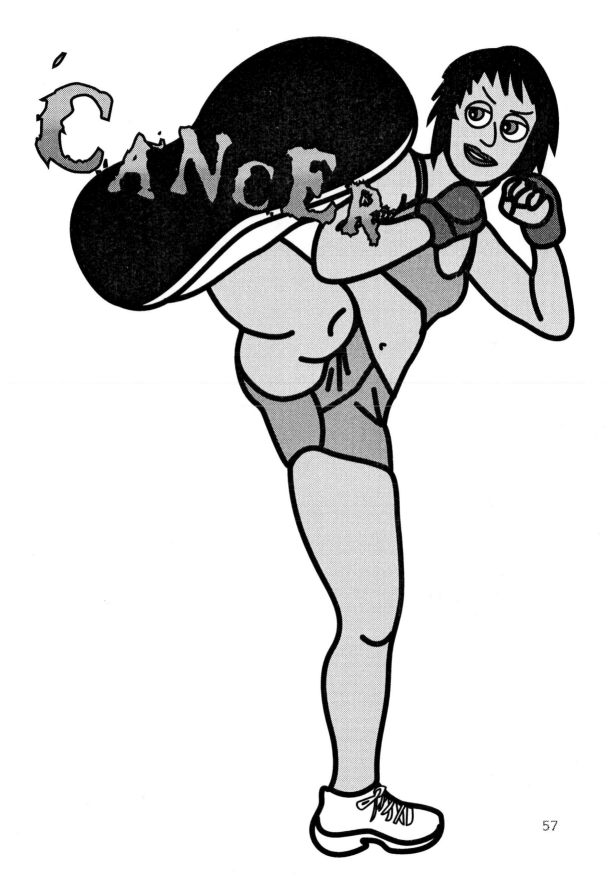

57

I just forgot what I wanted to tell you

**COMMON SYMPTOMS OF THE PHENOMENON
CALLED CHEMO BRAIN:**
- *The mental fog* (as described in my story on the next page)
- *Difficulty finding words*
- *Difficulty learning new information*
- *Difficulty completing tasks and multi-tasking*
- *Difficulty concentrating or focusing*

WHAT TO DO IF YOU EXPERIENCE CHEMO BRAIN:
- *Inform your oncologist* if you experience chemo brain. *Psychotherapy and medication can help.*
- Keep him/her informed about the *meds, special diets, and supplements you are taking*.
- *Use a single notebook to record everything* and date the pages. This way everything is in ONE place. Writing things down will free your mind and release stress.
- *Tape a checklist to your front door* to help you remember keys, wallet, cell phone, notebook, Cancer 101 planner, walk dog, lock doors, underwear (just kidding).
- *Use your Cancer101 planner*—write down things immediately, put them on your computer calendar, or leave yourself voice mail reminders.
- *Use a timer for cooking* and as a reminder to walk dog, pick up kids, etc.
- *Stay mentally and socially active* and tell others what's going on.
- *Eat healthy and exercise*—this helps your brain function.
- *Write down where you park your car* and how to get back to it.
- *Make a "home" at home for keys, glasses, cell phone, wallet*—a bowl on the kitchen counter.
- *Prioritize, simplify, rest, reduce stress, and give yourself a break.*

With all of the chemo and meds in your system, you may experience this condition. I certainly did. When I finished chemo, boy, did I feel different. Then I realized what a fog I had been in.

WARNING:
Some people experience delayed chemo brain. I know someone who encountered it two months after completing her chemo/radiation treatment. At least you'll know you're not going crazy. About 30% of people experience chemo brain. As always, talk to your oncologist and medical team. My chemo brain has improved daily. After all, I am writing this book.

— all about Chemo Brain

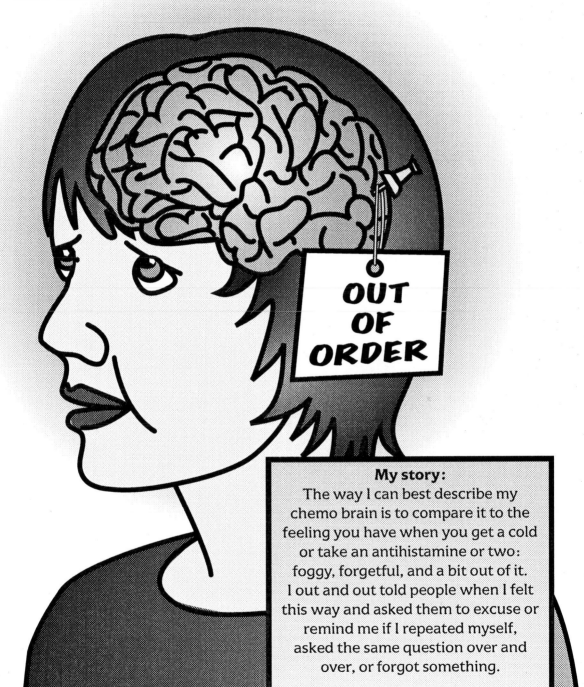

OUT
OF
ORDER

My story:
The way I can best describe my chemo brain is to compare it to the feeling you have when you get a cold or take an antihistamine or two: foggy, forgetful, and a bit out of it. I out and out told people when I felt this way and asked them to excuse or remind me if I repeated myself, asked the same question over and over, or forgot something.

Feeling DEPRESSED

AND WHO WOULDN'T BE?

We've all heard depression can result from a chemical imbalance. With everything you're going through and the chemicals/drugs going through you, you'll probably find yourself feeling depressed at some point before, during, or after chemotherapy. I did. Although this is a COMMON side effect, it can be a BIG deal, so I've devoted major space to the topic. I haven't met anyone who wasn't depressed at some point during chemo.

Many of our emotions relate to grieving for our loss of health, loss of control, loss of our normal looks, and loss of our routine.

THE FIVE STAGES OF GRIEF:
- *Denial*
- *Anger*
- *Bargaining*
- *Depression*
- *Acceptance*

SIGNS OF DEPRESSION—WHICH ALSO HAPPEN TO BE SIDE EFFECTS OF CHEMO:
- *Change in eating habits*
- *Change in sleep patterns*
- *Lethargy*
- *Anxiety*
- *Irritability*
- *Loss of concentration*

OTHER SIGNS OF DEPRESSION:
- *Loss of interest in usual activities*
- *Feelings of hopelessness*
- *Feelings of worthlessness*

IF YOU GET DEPRESSED (I DID), THEN GET SERIOUS:
- *Talk to your oncologist;* he may have suggestions, referrals and/or medications.
- *Talk to a psychotherapist*—insurance may cover this, or you may find a clinic that offers sliding scales and free services.
- *Take an anti-depressant* during this time with your doctor's approval and prescription.
- *Find a support group*—either in person, on the phone, or online.
- Seek help from your *spiritual community*.

IF YOU ARE FEELING DOWN:
- *Find a support group*—your spiritual community or cancer support group— either in person or over the phone.
- *Exercise*—a 30 minute walk outside in the fresh air can do wonders. Exercise can significantly decrease depression for everyone, especially those over 50.
- Get out of yourself and *help someone else*. I helped a friend with her resume. Make cupcakes for your neighbors who are giving you rides, write a thank you note, or send a birthday card. Swap favorite recipes with your neighbor. Teach someone something new on the computer.
- *Get lost in a good book, movie, play, or museum.*
- *LAUGH* at a funny movie, TV show, or comedian.
- *STOP reading cancer and chemo horror stories* on the Internet! Stop it!

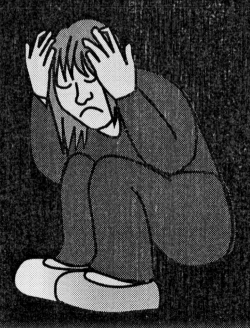

Make a list of what helps you rise out of

FOR ME, THE LIST LOOKS LIKE THIS:
- *Laughter* through friends, entertainment, the Internet, TV, movies, books, and magazines.
- *Doing something meaningful*—write or call someone you haven't talked to for a while. Give a gesture gift to neighbors who are giving you rides or cooking you meals. Something as small as a cupcake can be meaningful.
- *Getting together with friends.*
- *Getting outside the house*—walk outside and go to the coffee shop.
- *Attending my support group* at the Cancer Support Community.
- *Attending an easy exercise class* at the Cancer Support Community.
- Making my *gratitude list*.

STOP WORRYING:
Instead, gain knowledge and take action. Worrying takes up too much brain space. Worrying is a waste of time.
- *If you worry and something bad happens, you have suffered twice.*
- *If you worry and nothing happens, you have suffered once for no reason.*

OKAY. IF YOU INSIST ON WORRYING, DO IT DURING THE DAY AND NOT BEFORE BEDTIME:
- *Designate 15-30 minutes a day at a particular time for worrying. Then STOP!*
- *Try writing during this time. Putting worries on paper can help remove them from the brain.* Try brainstorming some solutions. If you're artistic and creative, convert your worry into a drawing, painting, or poem.

FEELING HELPLESS? HELP SOMEONE ELSE:
- *Helping my friend* Jocelyn (who can't drive) learn her local bus routes *gave me a different focus* and contributed to my sense of self-worth.

DAILY DO'S TO DIMINISH DEPRESSION:
- *A daily walk outside for fresh air*
- *A daily dose of laughter*
- *Daily, extend a kindness to someone. Yes, a smile will do.*
- *Daily gratitude list*

a downer day and then do those things

REMEMBER:
- *Do not identify with cancer. You are not your cancer.*
- *It is common for women in menopause to take anti-depressants*, because a change in hormones can create mood swings, feelings of hopelessness, powerlessness, and depression. ***Chemo may put you in menopause.***
- *Get help* from a friend, medication, support group, and/or psychotherapist.

WARNING:
If you do go on an anti-depressant, DO NOT just decide "Oh I'm feeling so much better and I don't need these." Do NOT just stop taking them. Consult your doctor. ***Stopping cold turkey is dangerous and may cause serious emotional fall-out and even psychosis.*** Ask your doctor for assistance to adjust your dose or wean you off anti-depressants.

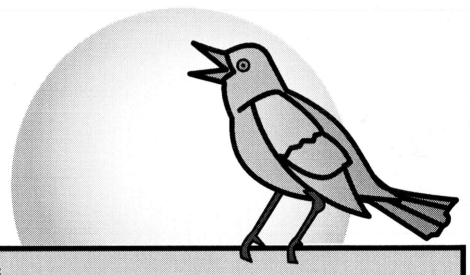

My story:
During this time I was prescribed a low dosage of an anti-depressant. I still felt like me, only I was less moody and didn't have so many meltdowns, crying jags, and feelings of being overwhelmed. I also attended a support group and learned tips I've included here. Plus I saw a psychotherapist, because my oncologist includes one on his medical team. That team consists of a surgeon, oncologist, radiologist, and psychotherapist. Great team!

Remember to be your own best friend

If you're still struggling with low energy, anxiety, and depression, do anything you can, however small, to make yourself feel better. At the same time, **when you're having a bad day, do not beat yourself up**. Self-blame is the last thing you need on top of everything else.

If all you can do is walk your dog for ten minutes, that's enough. If all you can do is pet your cat, that's fine for today. If all you can do is smile at your goldfish, no problem. If all you can do is hug your stuffed animal, okay. Some days are like that. Just don't let them go on and on. Remember, even baby steps to feeling good are still pointing you in the right direction.

HERE ARE A FEW REMEDIES

INSOMNIA:
- *Herbal teas, tryptophane, and melatonin* are natural remedies.
- *Exercise during the day*, but not within three hours before bedtime.
- *Prayer, meditation and visualization*
- *Relaxation CDs*, spoken word, nature, and white noise recordings
- *Relaxation and breathing techniques*
- *Prescription sleeping pills* from your oncologist. When I was taking steroids I needed a prescription sleeping pill to get to sleep. Sometimes just having the pill next to your bed helps, because you know it's there if you need it.
- *If you will be taking Tamoxifen post-chemo, take your pill in the morning,* because it may interfere with sleep.

ANXIETY:
- *Physical and meditative exercise* such as yoga, tai chi, and qui gong
- *Prayer and meditation*
- *Relaxation CDs*
- *Massage*
- *Animals*—pet your dog, cat, turtle (always wash your hands afterwards)
- *Nature*—lie in the grass and look up at the sky
- *Get creative*—paint, draw, garden, do craft
- *Soothing music*
- *Prescription anti-anxiety pills* from your oncologist

and lighten your load

RID YOURSELF OF RESENTMENT
- ***Don't allow someone who has hurt you to rent so much space in your mind.*** Use your mind for good things.
- ***Let go of anger, resentment and grudges.*** These feelings poison you instead of the transgressor.
- ***Forgive, let go and move on.*** Living well is the best way to get even!

That's right—forgiveness is the best revenge. Otherwise, someone is continuing to hurt you.

WHAT FORGIVENESS IS AND ISN'T
Dr. Fred Luskin, the author of *Forgive For Good*, was quoted in The Christopher's book, *Light One Candle*:
- Why do we allow someone who's nasty to us to rent so much space in our minds? Why?
- When you dwell on how someone has hurt you, you can forget what forgiveness is NOT.
- Forgiveness is ***NOT condoning, excusing, forgetting, or denying a wrong***.
- Forgiveness does ***NOT mean continuing a relationship, marriage, friendship, or work that is abusive***.
- Forgiveness is ***acknowledging that you've been hurt***.
- After that, forgiveness means ***giving up resentment***.

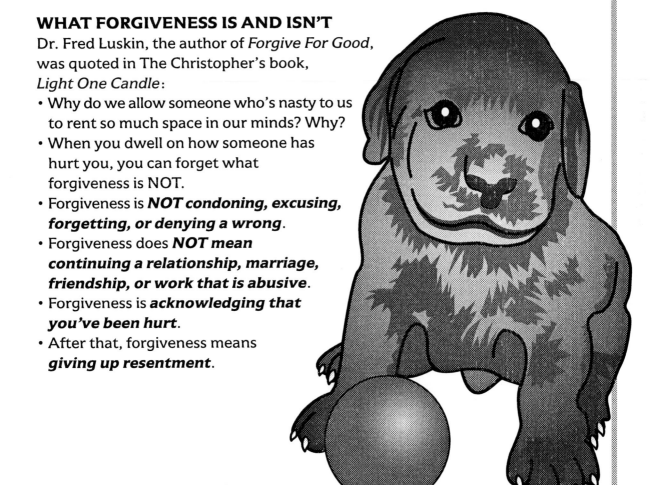

Can you pass the forgiveness final exam?

THE FINAL STEP IN HEALING YOURSELF—PER DR. LUSKIN:

- To be compassionate with the person who has hurt you is the result of much patience toward self and much prayer for the offending party.
- Practice forgiveness now. ***Your blood pressure will lower, your mood will be happier.***
- To forgive is to set the prisoner free and discover the prisoner was you!
- Forgiveness takes strength, courage and wisdom.
- ***Forgiveness empowers you!*** Forgiveness is real power!

My story:

I did use all the help available to me: psychotherapist, anti-depressant, support group, bosom buddy, exercise, daily walk, and my list as noted previously. Now, I feel I'm the best me I've ever been. And yes, I did manage to forgive a few people and move on. The best revenge is to forget the incident/people/institution and move on. This is so freeing and feels so good. If you don't do this, "they" get to keep hurting you. Don't let them do that. Really, I mean it!

Plus, I found that carrying on with my regular life in a modified version was great for alleviating depression. I had a good teacher. My friend Stella, who had colon cancer, continued to go out to plays, movies, and dinners with friends throughout her treatment. She fell asleep during these outings quite regularly. And, oh yes, she putted.

No one cared. Weird things happen with chemo, but people understand. She felt much better than sitting at home. Following her lead was a great choice for me.

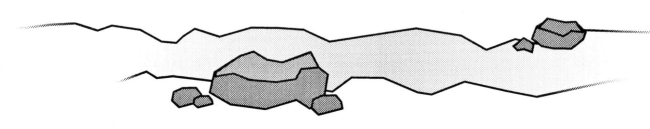

REMEMBER TO TAKE CARE OF THE CAREGIVER

Give the caregiver time off from his/her responsibilities. You may be the one going through treatment, *but your loved ones are also feeling stress, anxiety, and fear*. Let them know it's okay to enjoy life. They need to continue doing things that give them energy, joy, relaxation, comfort, and laughter. They need to eat healthy food, exercise, and keep up their social network. If they don't take care of themselves, how can they help take care of you? Caregiver support groups are beneficial, or your caregivers might wish to talk with a psychotherapist. They can get medications. They can get help on line, on the phone, or in person.

The Monks' Story

Two monks were travelling and came to a river. There they found a beautiful woman who was afraid to cross the rushing waters. The elder monk picked the woman up, despite his vows not to look at or touch women. He set her down on the other bank and continued along the road with his fellow monk. After a good distance, the companion could no longer contain his anger. "How could you break our vows and carry that woman?" the younger monk asked. The old monk replied, "I put her down hours ago, but I see that you are still carrying her."

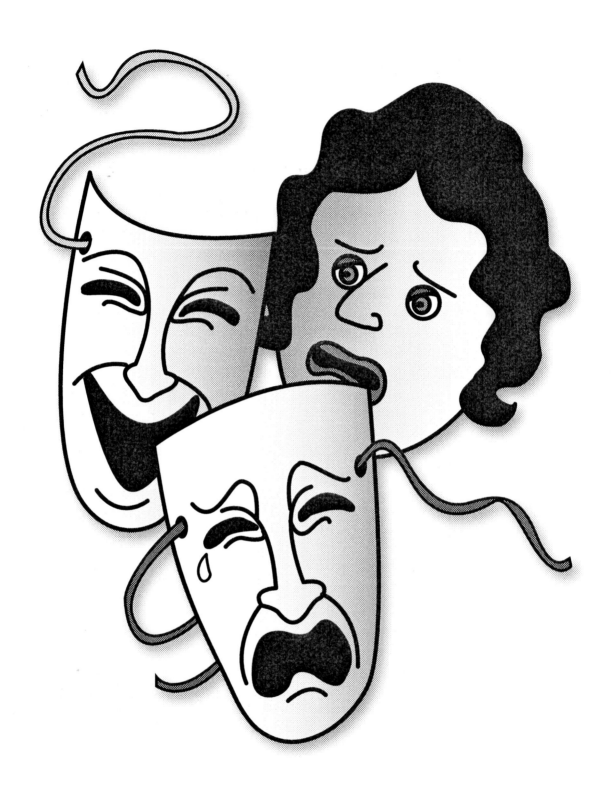

Post chemo highs and lows

Believe it or not, once your treatment ends you may find yourself depressed. This happened to me and **this is considered normal**.

DR. SUSAN LOVE, M.D., AUTHOR OF *DR. SUSAN LOVE'S BREAST BOOK,* DESCRIBES IT LIKE THIS:

"You're experiencing separation anxiety because the experience and preoccupation you've lived with so intensely is over. The routine established during your treatment has helped you feel supported, protected and active against your cancer. Losing that feeling is hard. It's a little like leaving a job—even one you didn't like. Rationally, you're glad it's over, but emotionally you feel lost." Dr. Love finds this one of the most helpful times for a woman to get involved with a support group. I agree. This is when I religiously went once a week to my support group.

The support group and exercise classes at my local Cancer Support Community helped me tremendously. I met women of all ages, ethnicities, religions, with all types and stages of cancer—in all phases—from just diagnosed, to out for years. My new friends gave me a wealth of advice, comfort, and many points of view.

When you feel fatigued, rubbery, and stiff with no hair and weird nails, no one understands how that feels like another woman who has gone through the same thing. Best of all, the support group provided laughter, friendship, and camaraderie. No, you don't cry, cry, cry at the support group. Yes, tears are shed and accepted, but I found that laughter, love, and joy far outweighed the tears. Plus the wonderful tips—many are in this book.

My support group taught me to begin coming back with small steps when chemo ended. I began to make a comeback. Stretching classes and that 30-minute walk outside started me on the physical road to recovery. And the support group gave me the emotional foundation to get on with my new life.

Rebirth and renewal

YES, THIS IS WHEN GOOD THINGS HAPPEN

My friend Christine calls this the rebirth glow. *You will know when you have it, and so will others.*

Now that you're feeling better and made it through the process, you'll find yourself looking forward to what's next. *Surprisingly, you may find that cancer is about living!*

Hopefully you've recognized that our time on planet Earth is limited. Knowing this can be a good thing. More importantly, you may have learned to treat yourself (and others) with loving kindness.

YOU MAY FIND YOU NOW RECOGNIZE YOUR PRIORITIES AND WANT TO SPEND AS MUCH TIME AS POSSIBLE . . .
- *doing what you want,*
- *with whom you want,*
- *when you want,*
- *where you want.*

While you're ridding your body of toxins, you may also want to rid yourself of toxic people. This includes the ones who drain your energy and are negative—the doomsday types. Dr. Judith Orloff's book *Emotional Freedom* can help you with this. Seriously!

YOU MAY HAVE LEARNED HOW TO:
- *focus on you.*
- *treat yourself with loving kindness.*
- *implement the honesty policy with loving kindness* (this does NOT mean brutal honesty).
- *be more compassionate, especially to those with illness or disabilities.*
- *ask for what you want, knowing other people can't read your mind.*
- *say NO.*

SAYING NO

Many of us have a difficult time saying "no." This can lead to doing things we don't want to do, then feeling angry and resentful. Stop it! Here's a tip: **You can simply say it: "No." Or pause and say, "Let me get back to you. Let me think about this. Let me check with my partner. Let me check my calendar."**

It's better to say "no" first and then later surprise people and say "yes" at the last minute. When you say "yes" and change that to "no," you often find yourself with unhappy, disappointed, and frustrated people. Who wants to lay that on others? However, you don't have to explain your "no." Oh, the wisdom I have gained through experience!

CHANGE CAN BE GOOD

Like many women, I had fun during rebirth and renewal. I changed my hair color, changed my work, rearranged my furniture and art, and uncluttered my house and life. Gee, you'd think I was still on steroids!

THE KORU

We began our book with the koru symbol and we end with the koru symbol. As Suzanne, a chemo recipient from our focus group, said: "The koru symbol is KEY to the entire book. It offers hope, meaning, and something to strive for and understand as you take the step by step journey through chemo, come out on the other side, and embrace the quest for new life, renewal, strength, love, and more."

We wish you everything the koru symbolizes!

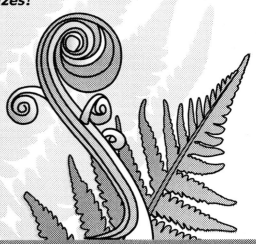

About Dr. Link

John Link, M.D. is recognized as one of the foremost breast cancer doctors in the world.
He actively practices at Breastlink, the comprehensive breast cancer group he founded in 1995. He also conducts research, writes books and teaches. The Breastlink Medical Group has been recognized as a leader and innovator in breast cancer care by *Self* magazine and ABC's *20/20*. In 1998, Dr. Link founded the Breast Cancer Care and Research Fund, a nonprofit charity dedicated to educating and helping women achieve optimal care. He has been recognized by numerous organizations for his dedication and contributions to women with this disease.

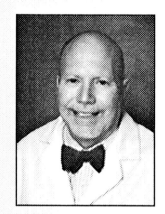

Dr. Link is the author of *The Breast Cancer Survival Manual* in its fifth edition and *Take Charge of Your Breast Cancer*. He has been honored by the American Cancer Society for his commitment to the treatment and cure of breast cancer.

About the authors

Roxanne Brown has a B.S. in business and has worked in sales, marketing, and management in the international home video field and advertising space sales. Later in life she returned to school and earned her M.S. in counseling, with an emphasis in career counseling. She's traveled extensively and has lived in the Midwest, on the East Coast, the West Coast, and in Europe. She now combines her education, experiences, and international contacts in her private practice and her contract work as a career counselor.

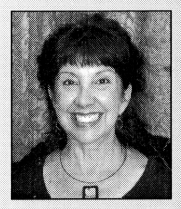

Roxanne is currently devoting her energy to promoting the positive benefits of _Chemo: Secrets to Thriving_ and is available to do presentations and book signings. She welcomes your comments and requests regarding the book and can be reached at roxCS2T@gmail.com.

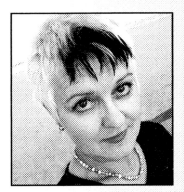

Designer and illustrator Barbara Mastej received a BFA from The School of Art at The University of Michigan, Ann Arbor, but has called Venice, California her home for over 25 years. Although she has spent most of her adult career working in both print and broadcast at large advertising agencies in Detroit, New York, and Los Angeles, she is currently half of a team in a creative partnership, Odd Man Out, LLC, with her mate and fellow artist, John Ransom. Her background in design, writing, and marketing is an invaluable tool for helping manifest ventures such as this book.

Barbara recently returned to her fine arts roots. Her paintings and other artwork can be seen at www.barbaraofvenice.com. Her design and advertising portfolio for Odd Man Out can be viewed at www.oddmanout.biz.

Acknowledgments

Special thanks to John Link, M.D., his new patient coordinator Stefany Montalbano, and the Breastlink Medical Group, whose energy directly propelled this project forward. One of the foremost breast oncologists worldwide, Dr. Link was so enthused when he saw the prototype of Chemo: Secrets to Thriving that he agreed to collaborate with us and requested a focus group study be done at his oncology center in Southern California. He surmised that "Chemo: Secrets to Thriving would increase the quality of life for people as they go through chemotherapy." I am eternally grateful for his help both as my personal physician and as a consultant on this book.

Thank you to the physicians, nurses, mental health professionals, patients, and caregivers who participated in our focus group. Thanks to the Cancer SUPPORT Community and HEALing Odyssey. These two organizations did SUPPORT and HEAL me. You can read about them in our Resources section.

Both my surgeon Dr. Steiner (the Michelangelo of breast surgery at Saul & Joyce Brandman Breast Center, Cedars-Sinai) and his assistant Susie Marble were huge cheerleaders and supporters. Susie also wanted this book out ASAP so she could give it to their patients. Susie's voice, manner, knowledge, and attitude first calmed me as I began my search for a surgeon. I'm so glad she was there and that, through her, I came to meet Dr. Steiner. Thanks Susie and Dr. Steiner!

I also want to thank my fellow chemo travelers who shared much of their knowledge, know-how, and insights, which greatly enhanced this book.

Thanks to Rosanne Lurie, who I met doing gentle yoga at the Cancer Support Community and who assisted in writing the Chemo and Financial Help section. Thanks Rosanne!

Thanks to Susie Chapperone who celebrated her end of chemo by getting married and assisted in writing our mouth sore section. She discovered new remedies and shares them right here, in this book. Susie and her caregiver husband Mark participated in our focus group. They encouraged me to keep soliciting agents and publishers by sending monthly e-mails: "When is the book coming out? We want it NOW to give to EVERYONE going through chemo!" Thanks Susie and Mark!

Emily Marsh introduced me to familypatient.com when her mother Jocelyn had a brain aneurysm. Jocelyn and Emily are doing fine now. Familypatient.com was so helpful during Jocelyn's three weeks in ICU, then the hospital, then a rehab home.

A big thank you goes to our cheerleader, editor, and financial supporter Steve Brown.

From its inception, our project manager John Ransom kept us true to the original intent and ensured the book became a reality.

Polly Ross, our editorial consultant, provided research and invaluable support during the search for a literary agent.

Krista Goering, our agent, found a unique publisher who was willing to embrace this unorthodox treatment of a medical theme.

Dee and Sammie Justesen at Norlights Press instantly "got" the book's concept and helped us finesse the content while preserving the book's quirky attitude by granting us creative license during the editorial process. Nadene Carter gave us guidance during the production process.

And finally, loving thanks to my dear friend Stella Fenton, who demonstrated what it means to thrive throughout her chemo treatment for colon cancer. In between traveling to San Diego from London to see her family, and attending movies, plays, museums, and greyhound races, Stella shared her own chemo secrets with me and inspired the title of this book. Thank you, Stella!

Roxanne's favorite resources

- *Organization kits and cancer information*
  www.cancer101.org • 1-646-638-2202

- *Blog (for free)—a healthy, fun way to communicate*
  www.familypatient.com
  www.caringbridge.org
  www.blogger.com

- *Career/work/health insurance information*
  www.cancerandcareers.org—get your FREE Living and Working with Cancer
  Workbook. This publication provides much information, resources and
  websites. www.patientadvocate.org • 1-800-532-5274
  www.healthinsuranceinfo.net

- *Scheduling help—making a meal, getting a ride or a baby sitter*
  www.lotsahelpinghands.com
  www.carecalendar.org

- *Look Good Feel Better · 1-800-395-5665*
  www.lookgoodfeelbetter.org helps cancer patients cope with appearance-
  related side effects of treatment. It's wonderful. I attended their local workshop
  and got a FREE tote with some free great makeup. Contact them!

- *Increase your energy and wellness—physically, mentally, financially,
  spiritually and more with The Cancer Support Community*
  www.cancersupportcommunity.org • 1-888-793-9355 provides education,
  hope, and physical and emotional support for people with all types of cancer
  and their loved ones. They offer on-line communities for patients, caregivers,
  and teens. I attended their exercise and art classes, lecture series, support
  groups, and more—all free of charge—even free parking in Los Angeles.
  This is one of the best things I did for myself. They were there for me (and they
  can be there for you) from beginning to end and beyond.

MORE GREAT RESOURCES:

- ***American Cancer Society**® · www.Cancer.org · 1-800-227-2345*
  ***For information about every major type of cancer**, email them or call
  the 24-hour telephone hotline where trained specialists will answer cancer-
  related questions, link you to resources, and inform you of local events.
  Services are available in English, Spanish, and other languages.

- ***CancerCare**® · www.CancerCare.org · 1-800-813-4673*
  Provides free, professional support services to anyone affected by cancer,
  including people with cancer, caregivers, children, and loved ones. Staffed by
  professional oncology social workers, CancerCare helps with many issues,
  including finding rides, financial help, applying for Medicaid, how to tell your
  child or boss you have cancer, what questions to ask your doctor, how to find
  a clinical trial, and more.

- ***www.ChemoAngels.net***
  Here's where you can connect with your own angel who will provide
  personal support throughout your treatment.

- ***Cleaning For a Reason** · www.CleaningForAReason.org*
  Free cleaning services for patients.

- ***Financial help can be found on pages 14-15 and also at:***
- ***www.patientadvocate.org** · 1-800-532-5274* and
  www.healthinsuranceinfo.net

- ***www.HeadCovers.com** · 1-800-264-4287*
  for comfy head covers.

Resources—continued

- **Learning to Forgive** · www.LearningToForgive.com
  Nine steps to forgiveness and more.

- **www.MyOncoFertility.org** · **1-866-708-3378**
  For answers to questions regarding cancer and fertility and pregnancy.

- **National Cancer Institute** · www.cancer.gov · **1-800-422-6237**
  The U.S. government's principal agency for cancer research.

- **Pregnant with Cancer** · www.PregnantWithCancer.org · **1-800-743-4471**
  Dedicated to **providing information, support, and hope to women diagnosed with cancer while pregnant**.

- **TeamSurvivor** · www.TeamSurvivor.org
  A great source for **exercise, health education, and support programs for women affected by cancer**.

- **TLC Direct** · www.tlcdirect.org · **1-800-850-9445**
  Provides online and/or direct mail catalogue with **wigs, hats, nightcaps, mastectomy products, and more for women going through chemo and cancer**. They are a not-for-profit affiliate of the American Cancer Society.

- **Young Survival Coalition** · www.YoungSurvival.org · **1-877-972-1011**
  Dedicated to the **concerns and issues that are unique to young women with breast cancer**.

NOTE: Many more resources are available to you. Ask your medical team, fellow chemo travelers, support group people, and check the resource lists in back of the books I recommend. Don't forget to check your local library.

Roxanne's favorite supplements

Not all supplements and remedies are successful or healthy for everyone.
EACH PERSON SHOULD CONSULT HIS OR HER DOCTOR BEFORE
TAKING ANY SUPPLEMENT OR REMEDY.

- *Floravital® Iron+Herbs—*
  liquid non-constipating iron supplement (pages 55-56)

- *Colon Helper™ BLF—*www.hcbl.com
  I take one in the p.m. for a soft bm in the morning—with my doc's okay.
  Ordered from Health Center for Better Living—800-544-4225. (page 52)

- *Trader Joe's blueberry or apple/cranberry fiber mini cakes—*
  breakfast muffins with added fiber

- *Glutamine Powder—*
  for throat sores and mouth sores (page 42)

- *Vitamin B6—*
  to help the healing process of oral tissue (page 42), help with
  neuropathy (page 51), and to boost your overall energy level (page 56)

- *Lysine—*
  for prevention of oral lesions (page 42)

- *Arm & Hammer® Baking Soda and Peroxide toothpaste —*
  gentle to your mouth and gums during chemotherapy (page 42)

- *Biotene® Mouthwash—*
  great for dry mouth and part of my mouth sore prevention remedy (page 42)

- *Claritin-D® 12-hour and/or Claritin-D® 24-hour—*
  remember, your doc must approve this, because it may be dangerous for
  some people. Claritin worked for my runny nose and relieved my bone
  pain (pages 30-31).

- *RevitaLash®—*
  to get eyelashes growing in thick and long (page 21)

FAVORITE SUPPLEMENTAL RETREAT:

- *Jumper cables for body, mind and spirit—take The Healing Odyssey*
  *www.HealingOdyssey.org · 1-949-951-3930—*provides a life altering
  (in the best way according to me) weekend. Provides practical tools, skills building,
  support, and humor to help you cope effectively with the effects of a cancer
  diagnosis and treatment. This is one of the best things I've ever done!

Roxanne's favorite books and

- John Link, M.D., *The Breast Cancer Survival Manual,* 5th Edition (New York, NY, Holt, Henry & Company, Inc., 2011)

- John Link, M.D., *Take Charge of Your Breast Cancer: A Guide to Getting the Best Possible Treatment* (New York, NY, Holt, Henry & Company, Inc., 2002)

- Susan M. Love, M.D. with Karen Lindsey, *Dr. Susan Love's Breast Book* (New York, NY, Da Capo Press, 2010)

- Dede Bonner, Ph.D., *The 10 Best Questions for Surviving Breast Cancer* (New York, NY, Simon & Shuster, 2008) My opinion—great questions for dealing with any cancer.

- Kim Thiboldeaux, Ph.D. and Mitch Golant, *The Total Cancer Wellness Guide: Reclaiming Your Life After Diagnosis* (Dallas, TX, Benbella Books, Inc., 2007)

- Kris Carr, *Crazy Sexy Cancer Tips* (Guilford, CT, Skirt! Books, 2007)

- David Chan, M.D., *Breast Cancer: Real Questions, Real Answers* (New York, NY, Marlowe and Company, LLC., 2006)

- Judith Orloff, M.D., *Emotional Freedom* (New York, NY, Crown Publishing Group, 2010)

publications

- Robert Maurer, Ph.D., *One Small Step Can Change Your Life: The Kaizen Way* (New York, NY, Workman Publishing Company, Inc., 2004)

- Rachel Naomi Remen, M.D., *Kitchen Table Wisdom: Stories That Heal* (New York, NY, Penguin Group U.S.A., 2006)

- Fred Luskin, Ph.D., *Forgive For Good: A Proven Prescription for Health and Happiness* (New York, NY, Harper Collins Publishers, 2003)

- Don Miguel Ruiz, *The Four Agreements: A Practical Guide to Personal Freedom* (Carlsbad, CA, Hay House, Inc., 1997)

- Go to www.copingmag.com to get *Coping With Cancer* magazine— 1-615-791-3859

- Go to www.AWomanshealth.com to get *Women Magazine* for information on health, wellness, prevention, treatment, community and cancer.

References

Brody, Jane E., *Family Planning When Cancer Intrudes*
(New York Times, Science Times April 21, 2009)

Brown, Zora K., Freeman, Harold P., MC with Platt, Elizabeth. *100 Questions & Answers About Breast Cancer Second Edition* (Sudbury, MA: Jones & Bartlett Publishers, Inc., 2007)

Carr, Kris, *Crazy Sexy Cancer Tips* (Guilford, Connecticut: Skirt! Globe Pequot Press, 2007)

Chan, David, MD., *Breast Cancer: Real Questions, Real Answers*
(New York: Marlowe & Company, 2006)

Cooper, Teri, *The View from the IVth Floor*
(*Women and Cancer* magazine, Fall 2007, pages 78-79)*

Cosmetic Executive Women Foundation, *Living and Working With Cancer Workbook*
(Roche Pharmaceuticals, 2007)

Link, John, M.D., Culllinane, Carey M.D., Kakkis, Jane M.D., Waisman, James M.D., *The Breast Cancer Survival Manual Fifth Edition* (New York: Owl Books, Henry Holt and Company, LLC., 2011)

Link, John, M.D., *Take Charge of Your Breast Cancer* (New York, NY: Henry Holt and Company, LLC., 2002)

Love, Susan M., M.D. with Lindsey, Karen, *Dr. Susan Love's Breast Book 5th Edition* (Cambridge, MA: Da Capo Press., 2010)

Luskin, Dr. Fred, *Forgive For Good* (New York, NY Harper Collins Publishers, 2003)

*Teri Cooper's article gave me the best wig tip: "...wearing a wig is very different when you have hair and when you don't. I found salvation from the irritation the wig caused my skin by placing paper towels between my scalp and the wig to form a cushion to the scalp and absorb the perspiration. (If paper towel manufacturers only knew how thankful I was for the help!)"

Rapkin, Michelle, *Any Day With Hair Is A Good Day*
(New York, NY Center Street Hatchette Book Group, 2007)

Roan, Shari, *Studies Find New Methods For Curbing Nausea of Chemotherapy*
(Los Angeles Times, May 15, 2009)

Silverman, Dan, M.D., PhD and Davidson, Idelle, *Your Brain After Chemo*
(Cambridge, MA, Da Capo Press, 2009)

The Christopher's, *It's Better To Light One Candle: Three Minutes A Day*
(New York, NY, The Christophers, 2004)

Thiboldeaux, Kim, President and CEO, The Cancer Support Community; Golant, Mitch PhD,
Vice President, Research & Development, *The Total Cancer Wellness Guide:
Reclaiming Your Life After Diagnosis* (Dallas, TX: Benbella Books, Inc., 2007)

Tripathy M.D., Debu, Editor-in-Chief: CURE, *Cancer Resource Guide Cancer Updates,
Research & Education* (Dallas, TX, Cure Media Group, 2008)

Women & Cancer Magazine (Ketchum, ID—Omni Health Media LLC—Summer 2009)

Breastlink Matters (Breastlink Newsletter, Orange, CA)

Other sources included my support group people and other thrivers I met at
The Cancer Support Community and The Healing Odyssey, people in the chemo room,
and even strangers who happened to sit by me.

Shopping List—things you may need:

GET THESE NOW—with your doc's okay— so you'll be prepared

- [ ] Organization kit from Cancer101.org (646-638-2202)
  - [ ] Calendar
  - [ ] Notebook or journal
  - [ ] Folders or accordion file

- [ ] Wig
- [ ] Metal brush
- [ ] Scarves
- [ ] Hat
- [ ] Paper towels (for under the wig)
- [ ] Nightcap (to keep head warm): www.Headcovers.com · 1-800-813-4287 or www.tlcdirect.org · 1-800-850-9445
- [ ] Claritin-D® 12 and/or Claritin-D® 24 (only if your doc says it's safe for you)
- [ ] Arm and Hammer® Baking Soda and Peroxide Toothpaste
- [ ] Biotene® Mouthwash
- [ ] Glutamine Powder
- [ ] Vitamin B6
- [ ] Lysine tablets
- [ ] Colon Helper™ BLF 1-800-544-4225 www.hcbl.com

- [ ] Florivital® Iron + Herbs liquid (non-constipating iron supplement)
- [ ] Ginger ale and salty pretzels (for nausea)
- [ ] Pickled ginger (Japanese store), ground ginger, ginger root (for nausea)
- [ ] Mint or ginger tea (for nausea)
- [ ] Lip balm/Carmex®/ChapStick® (for dry lips)
- [ ] Cornstarch/talcum powder for sore butt and underarm deodorant
- [ ] Tom's® Natural Deodorant
- [ ] Neosporin®/Vaseline®/Vicks VapoRub® (for dry nose)
- [ ] Soft facial tissues (for runny nose and runny eyes)
- [ ] Udderly Smooth® Udder Cream (800-345-7339) for dry skin or www.udderlysmooth.com
- [ ] Favorite music and movies*
- [ ] A selection of good books & magazines*
- [ ] Comfort foods that are easy to digest (Don't OD on sugar, as it depletes energy)
- [ ] Laughter stash
- [ ] *Living and Working With Cancer* **FREE** from www.CancerAndCareers.org

*Remember to use your local library and wash your hands after handling public materials.

Notes and advice from your doctor